Eat Well and Feel Great

Eat Well and Feel Great

The Teenager's Guide to Nutrition and Health

Tina Lond-Caulk

GREEN TREE
LONDON · OXFORD · NEW YORK · NEW DELHI · SYDNEY

Thank you to my darling husband Andy for your unfaltering support and encouragement. This book is dedicated to you, our beloved sons Ben & JJ and my dearest mother.

GREEN TREE
Bloomsbury Publishing Plc
50 Bedford Square, London, WC1B 3DP, UK
29 Earlsfort Terrace, Dublin 2, Ireland

BLOOMSBURY, GREEN TREE and the Green Tree logo are trademarks of Bloomsbury Publishing Plc

First published in 2021 in Great Britain as The Teenage Health and Wellness Guide

This edition published 2022

A catalogue record for this book is available from the British Library

Library of Congress Cataloguing-in-Publication data has been applied for

ISBN: TPB: 978-1-3994-0194-4; eBook: 978-1-3994-0192-0

4 6 8 10 9 7 5

Typeset in Ballinger by Deanta Global Publishing Services, Chennai, India
Printed and bound in Great Britain by CPI Trade (UK) Ltd, Croydon, CRO 4YY

To find out more about our authors and books visit www.bloomsbury.com and sign up for our newsletters

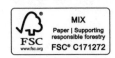

Contents

Foreword 6 ∗ Introduction 7

1. Set yourself up for success 9
2. Spot the signs of nutritional deficiency 17
3. Eat a rainbow and digestion 101 25
4. Fats won't make you fat (but they will make you smart) 39
5. Balance your blood sugar for all-day energy 47
6. Good hydration 54
7. What you eat can make you happier 62
8. Going plant-based 78
9. Love the skin you're in 87
10. Achieve a healthy weight for life 95
11. Gain weight and bulk up healthily 102
12. Teenage hormone imbalance 114
13. How to get more ZZZs 127
14. Build a healthy relationship with food 135
15. Managing your emotions around food 150
16. All about anxiety 158
17. Learning to love yourself 166

Quick and easy recipes 175

Further reading and resources 219 ∗ References 223
Glossary 232 ∗ Index 235 ∗ About the author 240

Foreword

As a nutritionist myself for over 20 years, I have witnessed first-hand the problems parents experienced raising their children, because their GPs had no nutritional information and 'domestic science' was abolished in many schools in the early 1960s. Even after I wrote *The Food Doctor for Babies and Children* in 2003, clients would call me in despair at the lack of readily available information to deal with weaning, teething, food intolerances and allergies, and my clinic was frequented by a plethora of young teens who simply wanted reliable information on everything from digestive disorders, skin problems and raging hormones to eating disorders.

Then along came the marvellous Tina Lond-Caulk (aka the Nutrition Guru), whose training and knowledge, determination and personal experience of motherhood have secured her place in the world of nutrition. She specialises in visiting schools up and down the country to deliver research-backed, informative lectures to students, teachers and parents alike, all in a digestible and simple-to-assimilate format. Alongside her presentations, she engages the students with practical work – the first hands-on approach for over half a century.

She has now collated the best of these teachings into the glorious book you hold in your hands and she has written it in a language that teenagers can understand, but which parents and teachers can be reassured has all been carefully researched and is backed up by published medical information.

At a time when the world is looking at significant issues such as sustainability, avoiding food waste, lowering fast food consumption and encouraging us all to cook real food for proper nourishment, this book could not provide better all-round support for the health and well-being of our next generation.

Tina, I salute you on such an engaging and expertly written book!

Vicki Edgson
Retired nutritional therapist

Introduction

This easy-to-use handbook is a guide on how to optimise your well-being so that you can achieve boundless energy and vitality, look and feel fantastic every day, and strive for all the things you want to do with your life.

Each year, I work with over 20,000 school students in my Food for Life education programme and over the last 20 years I've met hundreds of people in my busy clinical practice as an evidence-based nutritionist. Drawing on the combined power of these unique experiences, in this book I want to share my knowledge with you so that you too can realise the power that food and your daily habits have over your health and well-being.

I am hugely passionate about how nutrition and lifestyle habits affect every one of us, and have a first-class honours degree in nutrition and post-graduate training in eating disorders and behavioural psychology, as well as a special interest in nutrigenomics, which is the study of how nutrients affect your body's expression of your genes.

Through my work I meet many teenagers and young people who are struggling with health issues that are related to their understanding of nutrition, but also to their relationships with their bodies. So many people don't feel great when they first come to see me, but in a short time I get to see the rapid transformation in their energy levels, sleep quality, weight, mental well-being, skin health and confidence once they start taking better care of their incredible bodies.

Think of your body as a high-performance car. If you don't look after it and give it what it needs – fuel, oil, water and so on – it just can't perform. It simply won't work properly. You have a high-performance body that deserves the very best nutritional support. Without the right support you can start to feel sluggish, perhaps have low mood, develop skin issues, find it difficult to concentrate – the list goes on.

In this book you will learn how to develop a healthy and joyful relationship with your body and with food. You will learn how to spot the signs that your body needs specific nutritional support, as well as how to create harmony in your body and mind through healthy lifestyle habits and a balanced approach to your food choices. Most importantly, you can learn all about self-care. I look at all the topics that may be of interest to you as a teenager, from plant-based diets, skin health, muscle gains and improving your sleep, to building a healthy relationship with food and your body, and how to change some of your behaviours should you wish to. You can also learn how to maintain a healthy weight or indeed gain weight if that's what you need.

I hope this book inspires you to develop an understanding of how amazing your body is and what it needs to thrive. Create healthy habits and your body will reward you!

Chapter 1

Set yourself up for success

Do **you** want to enjoy...

- waking up feeling alert?
- loads of energy?
- a sharp mind?
- a balanced mood?
- good motivation?
- skin that glows?
- an effortless healthy weight?

You deserve to spring out of bed in the morning feeling totally recharged from a great night's sleep, full of energy, vitality and motivation to face each day. With this sense of wellness comes a great improvement in self-confidence too, and when you feel well, fit and strong you can achieve an enhanced sense of well-being.

I've worked with thousands of young people to help them feel fantastic, boost their confidence, increase their concentration and focus for their academic studies, improve their skin, hair and nails, and ensure they achieve a healthy weight and create a healthy, sustainable relationship with food. Every one of us deserves to feel well every day, both inside and out, and I'm going to show you how that's possible.

THE THREE STRANDS OF OVERALL GOOD HEALTH

Psychological health: sharp mind, good mood and motivation
Physical health: energy and ability to enjoy physical challenges, good sleep quality
Biochemical health: optimal levels of blood sugar balance, cholesterol, stress hormones and nutrient status.

The impact of what you eat

Food is information for our bodies. The chemical constituents in our foods literally tell our body how to behave, so what we eat can impact our moods, energy levels, motivation, ability to concentrate, to sleep and even whether we feel happy or sad.

Hopefully, we are all born in good health, but your lifestyle choices – your food intake, water consumption, how much you sleep, whether or not you exercise regularly and get proper relaxation and fresh air – will all affect whether or not you maintain that level of good health.

The following diagram shows a barometer of our health. Hopefully we are born with good health, giving us a high 'health deposit account'. However, depending on our dietary intake and lifestyle habits we can either stay in optimum health or move towards 'disease' and poor health, and we see changes such as those listed on the right-hand side. The first signs of someone being unhealthy are tiredness, sleep problems, low mood, low motivation, maybe getting coughs or colds, skin reactions or tummy problems. But you can reverse that, because our body loves to repair itself. Your bones can rebuild themselves in six weeks and, believe it or not, your skin is only 21 days old; that's ancient compared to your inner skin and gastrointestinal tract, which are just four days old, so if you burn the inside of your mouth, you will have new skin there in a mere four days.

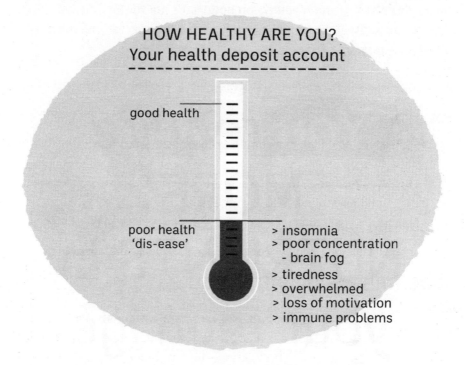

HOW HEALTHY ARE YOU?
Your health deposit account

good health

poor health
'dis-ease'

> insomnia
> poor concentration
  - brain fog
> tiredness
> overwhelmed
> loss of motivation
> immune problems

Your body is constantly recreating itself, so you can improve every aspect of your health and well-being. Don't worry about what habits you have had in the past – each day you can improve, starting today, so even if you're right down there in the red zone, in no time at all we can get you back to good health.

The basic idea of the 80:20 rule is very simple. In order to be healthy and balanced, you don't always have to make 100% healthy food choices.

The 80:20 rule

The 80:20 is an approach to healthy eating, teaching you balance, moderation and allowing for treats, without ever feeling guilty or worrying you are overindulging. There will be times when you need to be more flexible, like when you go on holiday or are having a celebration. This is absolutely fine and you can just get back to your balanced lifestyle afterwards.

You require MORE NUTRIENTS in your teenage years than at any other time in your life.

Making healthy choices 80% of the time is enough. For the remaining 20%, you can choose less healthy food and enjoy treat foods. Sometimes you will find that it will be 70:30 and that's just fine – being flexible and not rigid is vital for our overall relationship with food.

This will also help you stick to a healthier diet, because it's widely known that depriving yourself of all treats and sweets simply isn't sustainable, and can in itself create an unhealthy relationship with food or make an existing poor relationship even worse.

Let's talk about food

Before we look at what a healthier diet is, let's look at what you eat now. Do you eat a lot of junk food or ready meals, or do you order a lot of takeaways, without necessarily thinking about whether they're good for you or not, or what the alternatives are? I'm not judging, because I know it's easy to fall into a lifestyle where that's what you eat, but let's take a moment to consider some of the pros and cons.

JUNK FOODS – FOR OR AGAINST?

For	Against
Tasty	Lack the nutrients your body needs to function and thrive
Quick	Packed with unhealthy preservatives and additives
Convenient	Affect your concentration and academic performance
Cheap	Contribute to weight gain, obesity and disease
Hyper-palatable	Leaves you craving more and may gave you an insatiable appetite

In nature, we would never find foods that contain the combinations of high sugar, salt and fat found in ultra-processed and fast foods. These three compounds activate the pleasure and reward centre of our brain, leading us to want more and more, as our brain finds this mix truly addictive. This equation sums it up:

Sugar + salt + fat = the bliss point

The bliss point is where a particular food has just the right amount of saltiness, sweetness and richness to trigger a reward in your brain, in the form of a quick release of dopamine, triggering a kind of euphoria, bliss or feel-good vibe. Of course, this makes you feel good, so you subconsciously want to recreate that feeling by eating that particular food again. The combination of tastes is more rewarding than one of the substances acting on its own and it's the combination that produces the bliss point. This explains why ultra-processed and fast foods are so addictive.

When I talk about junk food, I'm referring to the foods that have very little or no nutritional value and contain high levels of fat, sugar, salt, refined seed oils and potentially additives and chemicals that your body doesn't like. Think of packaged snacks and meals like sweets, crisps, frozen pizzas, smoked bacon, chicken nuggets and sugary breakfast cereals. These are classified as unhealthy ultra-processed foods. Some foods are minimally processed but not unhealthy like bagged salads, roasted nuts, canned beans or tomatoes, frozen fruits, nut butter, tofu, milk, yoghurt (no added sugar) and hummus.

YOU ARE WHAT YOU EAT!

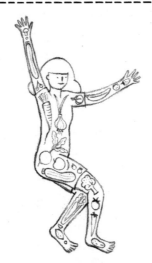

I regularly see young people in my clinic who are addicted to junk food, with the result that they feel sluggish, fatigued and may carry extra pounds. They may also have difficulty concentrating and have poor performance in school. In 2018, researchers at Manchester Metropolitan University looked at 11 existing studies, involving 100,000 participants aged 16 to 72, from Europe, the Middle East, the USA and Australia, and they found that 'a diet of fast food, cakes and processed meat increases your risk of depression'.

Certainly, if your diet is lacking in key nutrients or you are eating a diet that may cause inflammation, you are more likely to suffer low moods. In nutritional terms, inflammation is when the bacteria in our gut is altered and then interacts with our immune system, triggering it in a way that stimulates a response from the body. The swelling when you twist your ankle is a type of inflammation, but chronic inflammation can cause damage to cells, tissue and organs that may ultimately lead to health issues like diabetes or heart disease.

Junk food and ultra-processed foods have the ability to cause inflammation, but fortunately a healthy diet based on natural whole foods – natural foods with no added sugar, salt or fat – can also provide the building blocks for us to produce 'feel-good' neurotransmitters (the body's chemical messengers).

If you're someone who is always drawn to crisps, biscuits, burgers and fizzy drinks, I'm going to show you how some simple changes will make you feel great about yourself and get rid of those symptoms that may be niggling you. If you learn about healthy eating, the role of exercise, managing your stress levels and getting enough sleep in your teenage years, you're more likely to maintain these positive habits as an adult.

But before you embark on your road to optimising your health and well-being, it's important to know why you're doing it. Do you want to feel amazing, improve your mood, feel more energised or feel more confident in yourself? Once you find your why, it helps you keep on working towards that goal.

FINDING YOUR WHY!

Tick the things you want to improve

☐ Body confidence
☐ Daily energy balance
☐ Mood
☐ Motivation
☐ Focus
☐ Skin health
☐ Hair health
☐ Specific symptoms (such as headaches)
☐ Weight
☐ Sleep quality
☐ Other (give details) ....

✳ Summary ✳

What we eat has a major impact on how we feel and our overall well-being. Eating too many ultra-processed foods, including pre-packaged snacks (biscuits, chocolate bars, crisps and sweets), ready meals and takeaways, can leave us feeling tired, moody, unfocused or simply unwell. When we eat natural foods, our bodies absorb the nutrients efficiently and easily, so eating a healthy, balanced diet is the best way to achieve boundless energy, boost our mood and concentration, sleep better and, of course, prevent diseases in the future.

The human body is incredibly efficient at repairing itself, so even if you recognise you have some bad habits, you can change them and start improving your health right now. One effective approach is the 80:20 rule, which says that you can still live your best life if roughly 80% of your food choices are healthy and 20% are less healthy.

chapter 2

Spot the signs of nutritional deficiency

It's estimated that 40–50% of teenagers will have one or more nutrient deficiencies. This can affect how you feel and whether or not you truly thrive. Along with essential fatty acids (the fats we can't make in our bodies), four of the most commonly occurring nutrient deficiencies in the UK are iron, magnesium, calcium and omega-3.

So why are nutrition deficiencies so common in teenagers?

During the teenage years the body and brain are still developing, which creates an increased demand for key nutrients. Teenagers might also have a tendency not to plan what they eat, skip meals or rely on ultra-processed or pre-packaged foods. You can end up eating a very narrow range of foods and may decide to leave out some food groups altogether, such as carbohydrates, proteins or fats.

Our bodies have an extraordinary ability to show us when they need specific nutrients, so let's have a look at some of the symptoms that could be a sign you have a nutritional deficiency.

MATCH YOUR SYMPTOM...

Symptom	Possible nutrition deficiency or cause
Low mood	Vitamin D, Vitamins B6 and B12, essential fatty acids like omega-3 (every cell in our body needs them to function and we can only get them from our diet), iron, magnesium, zinc, iodine, selenium
Lowered immunity	Essential fatty acids, vitamins A, C, D and E, zinc, iron, selenium, copper, folate
Tiredness/fatigue	Iron, vitamins B, B12 and D, omega-3, magnesium, dehydration
Dry skin, dandruff, eczema	Essential fatty acids, vitamins A, D and E, zinc
Acne	Vitamin A, D and E, zinc, essential fatty acids
Muscle cramps	Magnesium, vitamins B and D, potassium
Poor concentration, memory and attention	Essential fatty acids, zinc, iron
Hair loss	Iron, vitamins A, B12, C, D and E, zinc, folate, biotin
Plugged hair follicles (small bumps under the skin)	Vitamin A, B, C and E, essential fatty acids

Dark circles under eyes	Iron, (dehydration or allergies)
Brittle, flaking nails	Iron, essential fatty acids, biotin, vitamins B12 and D, zinc
Sore tongue	Iron, vitamin B12, folate, niacin
White tongue	Gut bacteria imbalance, vitamin B
Burning sensation in tongue or feet	Vitamins B6 and B12, folate
Smooth tongue (very pale)	Iron
Swollen tongue	Iron, B vitamins
Mouth ulcers	Iron, vitamin B12, folate, iron, zinc
Numbness and tingling around mouth	Calcium, vitamin B12, folate, (allergies)
Cracking lips	Vitamins B1, B2, B3 and B12
Bone pain	Vitamin D
Excessive bruising	Vitamin C
Slow wound healing	Vitamins A, B, C and D, zinc
Constipation	Fibre, (or dehydration)
Irregular heartbeat	Calcium, magnesium

And to switch it round, if you do have one of the common nutrient deficiencies, here are some of the symptoms you might be experiencing.

Iron

Pale complexion
Dark circles under the eyes
Sore or swollen tongue
Headaches or dizziness
Poor concentration
Poor ability to learn and remember
Breathlessness
Heart palpitations
Brittle or spoon-shaped nails
Fatigue

Calcium

Low mood
Numbness or tingling in hands or feet
Muscle cramps
Fainting
Insomnia
Bone loss (bones fracture easily)
Delayed onset of puberty
Brittle or weak nails

Magnesium

Lethargy
Irritability and anxiety
Loss of appetite
Muscle cramps and spasms
Facial or eye twitches
Difficulty sleeping

Vitamin D

Low mood
Fatigue
Muscle weakness
Stiffness and achy bones
Poor immunity

> Think FOOD FIRST. Food is information: it informs our bodies how to behave and affects our metabolism, immunity and how we think and feel. If you aren't feeling 100%, upgrading your diet with nutrients can help improve your mood, energy, skin and overall wellbeing.

Mythbusters

To avoid nutrient deficiencies, we all need to eat a healthy, balanced diet. However, there are many contradictory messages around food, nutrition, health and weight, so let me dispel some of the myths I hear every day (in case you're wondering, the myths are in bold!).

- **There are 'good' and 'bad' foods.** Wrong! All foods can feature in a balanced diet. It's the quantity and frequency of foods that matters.

- **Carbohydrates are the enemy.** They're not. They are our body's and our brain's main source of fuel. They not only help us feel energised, but they can also keep us feeling full for longer and stop sugary food cravings. Complex carbohydrates can be a key player in maintaining a healthy weight and keeping our mood stable. They are a good source of a substance called tryptophan and when tryptophan enters your brain, more of the happy hormone serotonin is produced and your mood tends to improve. Carbohydrates are also great food for your gut and a happy gut makes more happy hormones too (see page 67).

- **Always count calories.** No, don't worry about that. Trust your hunger and fullness cues, and practise eating mindfully. Balancing your plate at each mealtime with the healthy plate layout (see page 32) will ensure you have stable energy levels and feel full up for longer, and won't get the blood sugar dips that drive hunger.

- **Vegetarian and vegan diets are always healthier.** Vegetarian and vegan diets can be healthy if they are rich in plants and include lots of whole grains, but they can also lack certain nutrients. By removing all animal products and fish from your diet, you may be lacking in protein, calcium, iron, iodine, choline, omega-3 fats and vitamin B12. You can find many of these nutrients in eggs and dairy if you're vegetarian, and in fortified products if you're vegan. Some meat replacement and vegetarian or vegan food products are highly processed with lots of additives and unhealthy ingredients, so read the labels and avoid foods that are over-processed. See Chapter 8 for tips on going plant-based.

- **Detoxing is important.** In fact, your body has a built-in detoxification system: your lungs and other organs work around the clock to remove harmful substances. Drink plenty of clean water, reduce your exposure to chemicals (pesticides, personal hygiene products, plastics), exercise (and sweat) regularly and, along with your daily bowel movements, that will ensure healthy detoxification.

- **Gluten-free is healthier.** There's little evidence to suggest gluten-free has any particular health benefits unless you are a coeliac or have a gluten intolerance. In fact, cutting out all foods containing gluten can be incredibly limiting and mean you consume far less fibre and nutrients in your diet, leading to gut health issues, including constipation. Gluten-free replacement foods often contain bulking and emulsifying chemicals with no nutritional value and they can lack all-important fibre. If you need to eat gluten-free because of a genuine medical condition, it is better to eat naturally gluten-free grains.

- **Sugar-free diet drinks and food are better for you.** The latest science shows that the artificial sweeteners in diet drinks and food disrupt our important gut microbiota and may lead to increased weight gain and type 2 diabetes. Sugar in moderation may be a safer choice as it is a 'real' food rather than a man-made, artificial product. Having said that, many commercial food products are laden with added sugars, so be careful not to overdo your sugar intake. Go ahead and enjoy the occasional sweet treat – head to page 211 for some recipe ideas.

- **If you're skinny, you're healthy.** In fact, just because you're thin it doesn't mean you're healthy, because a very slim person may be under-nourished. We can be healthy at every size. Rather than fixating on body shape or dress size, enjoy a nutritious diet and maintain an active lifestyle, as these behaviours often improve your body weight, lean muscle mass and body fat percentage.

- **You should compare your body to others.** We each come in a different shape and size, which is what makes us so interesting and beautiful, and we are also so much more than our body shape.

- **You need to eat like your friends.** You don't. You are unique. Your energy and nutritional needs will differ. Don't worry about following trends.

- **Fats make you fat.** Fats tend to have a bad rep, but healthy fats are a really important part of a balanced diet. They support brain health, keep our skin nourished, make sure we feel full for longer, are a great source of energy and help support hormone balance. You can learn more about healthy fats in Chapter 4.

- **Skipping breakfast is a good idea.** In your teenage years consuming breakfast is VERY important, so skipping breakfast or any other occasional fasting is a bad idea. Studies show that having breakfast improves concentration and mood, and ultimately academic outcomes, but opt for something that will release energy slowly (see the breakfast recipes on pages 176–183).

- **Snacking is bad for you.** If you get tired and hungry between meals then a healthy snack is a good idea. Just make sure you plan ahead and carry snacks with you so you make better choices and aren't tempted to buy processed snacks that are high in sugar and saturated fats.

- **Healthy food is really expensive.** It doesn't have to be! Although organic produce, unprocessed meat and fish, and nuts and seeds can be expensive, the basic elements of a whole foods diet (such as fruits, vegetables, legumes and grains) are affordable supermarket items. Buying in bulk, at local markets and at the end of the day in supermarket reduced sections is a great way to make food more affordable. Picking frozen meat, fish, vegetables and fruit are also cost-effective ways to eat well on a budget. To help remove pesticides from non-organic fruit and veggies, soak them in vinegar (any type) and water for 20 minutes. Aim for one part vinegar to four parts water.

- **Food is just fuel.** It is fuel, but it's also so much more than that. Good food nourishes our bodies and we should take pleasure in it. A beautifully presented meal is an instant mood-enhancer, so experiment and make your food colourful, varied and interesting. It's scientifically proven that food presentation makes food taste better too.

- **What you read about food and health is always true.** What do you think? Is it? The sensible approach is to check the source of the information. Who wrote it and what qualifications do they have? Do they have a degree in nutrition or have they just done a short online course? It takes years of studying to learn everything about nutrition and health.

TOP TIP

→ Aim for 30 different plant foods each week, including whole grains, fruits, veggies, nuts, seeds, herbs and spices. Try making smoothies with frozen fruits, green leaves, nuts and seeds; buy bagged salads with different leaves and top with mixed nuts, seeds and dried fruits; cook with fresh or dried herbs; or try a granola like Bio&Me which offers 15 different plants in one portion. ←

✳ Summary ✳

Although we have an abundance of food and calories in the UK, nutrient deficiencies are still very common, particularly among teenagers. If you recognise any of the symptoms listed in this chapter, you may have a nutrient deficiency. To maintain good levels of all nutrients, aim to eat a healthy balanced and varied diet. Variety ensures you get the widest range of nutrients you can. There are a lot of myths around about what a healthy balanced diet is, so make sure you know the true facts. Creating a weekly menu plan to ensure you are including all the key food groups is a great way to get started. To change your dietary habits, visualise yourself feeling energised, healthy, nourished, glowing and confident from eating well – associate your diet with health, happiness and energy.

chapter 3

Eat a rainbow and digestion 101

Did you know that eating more fresh fruits and vegetables can make you more attractive as they improve your skin tone and can make you glow? Yup, it's true. Google it!

The colours we see in plants are called phytonutrients. They protect plants from disease, and when we eat them, they also protect us from disease. The pigments that give fruits and vegetables their bright colours represent a variety of beneficial compounds. By eating all the colours of the nutrition rainbow, you'll harness these power-packed foods! A fun fact about food is explained by the term 'doctrine of signatures'. Food resembling various parts of the body can be used to heal those body parts. Here are some examples:

- Citrus fruits look like breasts and help keep breasts healthy by assisting lymphatic circulation, which filters out harmful substances and regulates fluid balance in breast tissue.

- A slice of carrot looks like a human eye and carrots contain lots of antioxidants, which protect the health of your eyes.

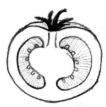
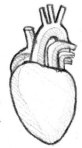

A tomato has four chambers and is red just like the heart. A tomato is loaded with lycopene, which is pure heart and blood food.

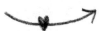

- A walnut doesn't just look like a brain, walnuts provide nutrients such as healthy fatty acids that specifically nourish our brain, help with memory and mental function, and stimulate the production of important neurotransmitters, including serotonin.

- A tomato has four sections, rather like the four chambers of the heart, and it contains a range of antioxidants and nutrients, including something called lycopene, which can help lower blood pressure and boost heart health.

- A bunch of grapes looks like blood cells and not only are they good for the blood, they boost brain power, and support eye and heart health too.

- Red kidney beans are kidney-shaped and they promote kidney health, plus they contain lots of soluble and insoluble fibre, which enhances cardiovascular health and helps keep your blood pressure low.

- A stick of celery looks like a bone and cracks just like a bone, and celery is good for strengthening bones, particularly if they've been damaged.

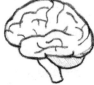

A walnut looks like the brain and helps develop more than three dozen neurotransmitters to enhance brain functions.

Eat the rainbow every day

Yes, eating a variety of colourful foods is good for your health, but how do you make that happen? Start by eating a beautiful breakfast. Start your day with a smoothie packed with fruit and veg, oats topped with red berries or an omelette filled with red peppers, mushrooms, spinach or other colourful veggies.

Continue the day with a lovely lunch in which vegetables are the star of the show. You could opt for soup or a sandwich packed with a range of brightly coloured veg or, even better, a large, colourful salad.

Whether it's at lunchtime or in the evening, aim to have at least one big salad every day, packing your plate with as many different variations on a vegetable theme as you can. The recipe section (see page 201) explains how you put together a Buddha bowl and has lots of other inspirational ideas too. Why not challenge yourself to create your own rainbow meal using every colour (white means vegetables like garlic, cauliflower, onions and potatoes, not sliced white bread!).

WHAT DIFFERENT COLOURS DO

Food colour	What phytonutrients in that food colour support
Red	Skin health, soaks up free radicals, heart health, cancer prevention
Yellow/orange	Eye health and vision, sun protection, immunity, heart health, cancer prevention
Green	Energy and vitality, healing, the production of digestive enzymes, detoxification, immunity
Purple/blue	Positive mood, memory, cell protection, anti-inflammation, cancer prevention , brain health
Brown/white	Anti-inflammation, heart health, cancer prevention, hormone balance, detoxification, lower cholesterol

So, to do all of the above, as well as maintaining a healthy weight, feeding your brain and aiding sleep, aim to eat a minimum of one fist-sized portion from each colour group each day to ensure you're getting the widest variety of healthy, protective, immune-supporting nutrients. Ideally, the goal is to eat between seven and ten fist-sized portions of different fresh fruits and vegetables every day. An ideal split is two to three fruits and five to seven portions of vegetables.

The whole spectrum

To make sure you're covering all colours of vegetable, fill in this checklist – see if you can get at least one tick in every column every day.

	Red	Yellow/orange	Green	Purple/blue	Brown/white
	Radicchio Radish Red lentils Red lettuce Red onions Red peppers Tomatoes	Butternut squash Carrots Orange peppers Pumpkin Squash Sweetcorn Sweet potatoes Yellow lentils Yellow peppers Yellow split peas	Asparagus Avocado Broccoli Brussels sprouts Cabbage Celery Green olives Green peppers Kale Pak choi Peas Watercress Rocket	Aubergine Beetroot Black olives Purple broccoli Purple carrots Purple potatoes Red cabbage	Cauliflower Chickpeas Fennel Mushrooms Onions Parsnips Shallots Turnips
Monday					
Tuesday					
Wednesday					
Thursday					
Friday					
Saturday					
Sunday					

Healthy portions

If you want to reach and maintain a healthy weight, first you need to check that you're eating a range of different foods and that you're eating the right number of portions of each one.

HOW MANY PORTIONS?

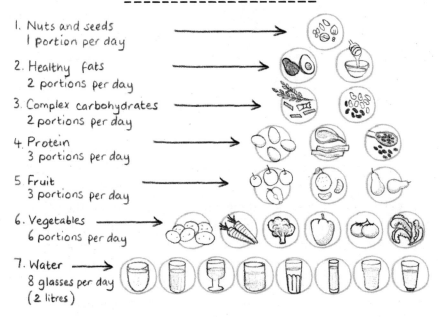

1. Nuts and seeds
   1 portion per day

2. Healthy fats
   2 portions per day

3. Complex carbohydrates
   2 portions per day

4. Protein
   3 portions per day

5. Fruit
   3 portions per day

6. Vegetables
   6 portions per day

7. Water
   8 glasses per day
   (2 litres)

Then you need to check that your portions are the right size. Aim to eat all the following food groups each day in the correct portion sizes.

Obviously, portion sizes vary depending on what you're eating, so one portion of salad leaves or a leafy green vegetable is two good handfuls, but if it's butter one portion is roughly what you could balance on a single fingertip. You can have a little more cheese or nut butter – about a thumb's worth – and a portion of protein will fill the palm of your hand (twice that if it's a plant-based protein like tofu). When you're talking about carbs, a portion is about the size of your fist, and you can fill a cupped hand with a snack portion of dried fruit, nuts or seeds.

WHAT MAKES A GOOD PORTION?

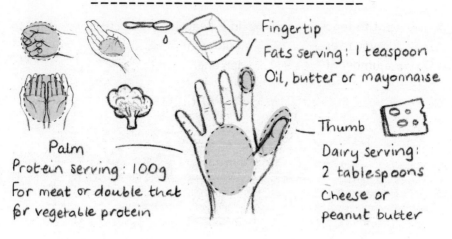

Fingertip
Fats serving: 1 teaspoon
Oil, butter or mayonnaise

Palm
Protein serving: 100g
For meat or double that
for vegetable protein

Thumb
Dairy serving:
2 tablespoons
Cheese or
peanut butter

You also need to check your plate size. Plate sizes are so much bigger than they used to be 50 years ago – along with waistlines! – so aim to eat from a plate that is no more than 25 cm in diameter. Visualising portions is far easier than weighing and measuring out your food. The rule for a healthy plate layout is 50% colourful fruit and vegetables, 25% protein and 25% complex carbohydrates, although if you're an active teenager, the balance should be more like 33% fruit and veg, 33% protein and 33% complex carbs.

Each plate should also include two teaspoons of healthy fats (that's six per day). All the following contain one teaspoon of healthy fats so you can mix and match:

- 1 tablespoon of olive oil
- 1 tablespoon of seeds
- ½ an avocado
- 1 ½ teaspoons of nut butter
- 8 large olives
- 30g of nuts

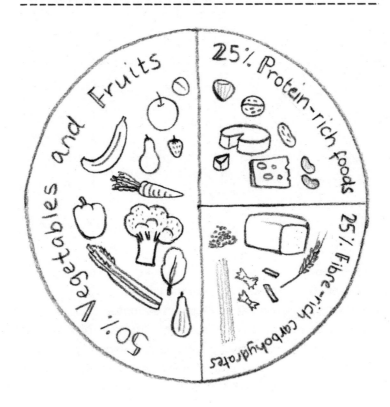

Digestion 101

Ultra-processed and greasy, high-fat foods can be very hard to digest, but even if you buy and eat the healthiest food in the world, if you don't digest it properly and absorb the nutrients, it won't do you any good.

When we are stressed, rushing about, we are in 'fight or flight' mode, which means our digestive functioning is on hold and we are unable to digest our food. Also, if we eat our food too quickly, we can't break it down effectively and take in the nutrients.

Try to sit up straight during and after a meal. If you slump or crash on a sofa straight afterwards, you're just squishing your poor, full stomach. I can't stress enough the importance of keeping hydrated, so drink water, but do it between meals. Sipping a little throughout a meal is fine, but avoid drinking large amounts just before, during and just after meals, because this can inhibit the digestive process.

To check whether you're making enough saliva, try eating a cream cracker. If you need water to wash it down, you're probably a bit short on saliva (and could be short on other digestive juices too), so up the quantity of water you're drinking in order to up your saliva production. Signs that you are not making enough saliva include: difficulty chewing, swallowing, dryness in your mouth, bad breath and a dry tongue.

TOP TIP

→ **If you're feeling stressed or have been running around, you need to switch off the stress hormones and switch on the digestive processes. Before you start to eat, take a few deep breaths. By pausing and focusing on your food you will trigger the 'rest and digest' mode, and breathing deeply is an excellent way to achieve this.** ←

The act of chewing stimulates the production of saliva, stomach acid and digestive enzymes, all of which are required to ensure your food is fully digested and the nutrients from your food are absorbed. Chew slowly and get that saliva working. You want all those chewy and chunky bits ground up and mixed with enough saliva to start digestion.

Chewing also helps you feel full after a meal, and this has been shown to reduce food cravings and stop us overeating, and stimulates peristaltic movement in your gut (the contraction and relaxation of muscles), which helps move your food through the system at the optimum speed and maintain blood sugar regulation so you don't feel tired after eating. This can help prevent symptoms such as indigestion and heartburn. What's more, the act of chewing has even been shown to reduce stress, which may also improve digestion.

It takes 20 minutes for your brain to realise that your stomach is full. Therefore, taking the time to eat slowly and pay attention to how full you're getting can help prevent common digestive problems and stop you overeating.

Regular exercise can improve digestion too. Exercise and gravity help food travel through your digestive system. A good rule of thumb is to wait up to 60 minutes after a small meal or two to three hours after a normal to large meal before exercising as otherwise it can leave you with stomach cramps. However, everyone is different, so see what works for you.

If you want to improve your digestion, try to develop the following good habits:

- Put your phone down and really focus on your food

- Concentrate on how it looks and smells

- Choose each mouthful carefully and chew it slowly

- Savour how each bite feels in your mouth and above all how it tastes

- Put your knife and fork down between each mouthful

- Don't drink a lot of fluids during a meal as this can stop good digestion

- Create time every day when you can go for a poo and don't have to rush.

In a study of people with chronic constipation, a daily exercise regimen including 30 minutes of walking significantly improved symptoms, which is good news for the one in a hundred young people aged between 11 and 18 years who have constipation. People who eat lots of processed foods, cheese, meat, white bread and bagels may find they're constipated more often, and the signs and symptoms of constipation include:

- Smelly farts and poos – and farting a lot

- Not doing poos very often

- Doing poos that are either massive or tiny pellets

- Discomfort or pain in your stomach

- Poor appetite

- Lack of energy

- Irritable, angry or miserable mood

- Skin issues, such as rashes, acne or spots

As well as getting more exercise to move food through your digestive system more efficiently, to avoid constipation drink more liquid throughout the day; eat meals at regular set times rather than skipping meals or eating at different times; and include more high-fibre foods in your diet – try apples, pears, oranges, ripe bananas, beans, oats, wholegrain breads and popcorn or add flax meal or chia seeds to homemade fruit smoothies. Most importantly, don't avoid the urge to go – if you do, it can make it harder to go later. However, you may be fearful of going to the toilet outside your own home, in which case you are not alone. Would you believe that this affects up to 32% of the population, men and women, to some degree? Understanding that we all need to visit the toilet frequently for our bodies to be healthy is key, but if you are struggling you should ask your GP for help as cognitive behavioural therapy (CBT) or hypnotherapy can both be helpful in overcoming this social anxiety fear.

Beat the bloat

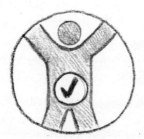

Feeling bloated after eating is part of normal digestion and is really nothing to fret about. When your body starts digesting what you've eaten, the carbohydrates break down and the fibre ferments, which produces gas. This then expands, causing bloating. Your core area might feel full, tight or gassy, or your stomach might stick out (some people call this a 'food baby'). Bloating can be relieved by farting, doing a poo, drinking a warm drink to relax the digestive system, doing some light stretching, or it just goes away in time as your food is digested.

Whole foods are healthy and I recommend they play a major part in your diet, but when you first start eating them you may find you're feeling bloated and getting excess gas, because your body may need to adjust to digesting them.

What causes bloating?

Foods that can cause bloating:

- Beans and legumes
- Cruciferous vegetables, particularly raw kale
- Fibre-rich chia and flax seeds
- Fibre-rich foods in general
- Fat-rich foods
- Sugar substitutes such as artificial sweeteners or xylitol
- Fermented foods such as pickles

Things that you may not know can cause bloating:

- Not chewing your food thoroughly – unchewed food, particularly carbohydrate, can't be digested and starts to ferment
- Eating too fast – for the same reason
- Eating large or oversized portions
- Not eating enough fibre
- Not drinking enough water
- Drinking fizzy drinks, including sparkling water
- Newly introduced probiotic supplements or fermented foods
- Taking certain medications, such as multivitamins, iron, antacids
- Not doing a poo at least once a day
- Feeling very stressed
- Smoking
- Eating too close to bedtime

Digestion begins in the mouth, so you need to chew each mouthful thoroughly, approximately 20 to 30 times, to ensure you digest the food you are eating.

Keeping the gut happy

If you need a little temporary relief to ease bloating, grab a cup of hot water with fresh mint or a peppermint tea (if you have acid reflux, opt for ginger instead), which can help soothe digestion and release gas. Then take a short five- or ten-minute walk, do some light core stretching and try to go to the loo if you can. Take five minutes of deep breathing to decrease stress, drink plenty of water and make sure you chew your food properly at your next meal.

Stress can also cause bloating by stimulating the body's fight or flight response, which negatively impacts gut health and impedes our digestion. So if you experience bloating, indigestion, flatulence, constipation, cramps or other gastrointestinal problems, it may well be worth investigating whether your emotions and stress levels might be contributory factors.

You might also find anxiety-relieving techniques such as breathing exercises, meditation or yoga, which you can learn and practise from apps, will help to relieve digestive problems, as well as relax you and help you sleep (for example, there's a well-known yoga move called wind-relieving pose that can shift bloating and gas).

How healthy is your poo?

We need to excrete our waste every day. If not, we start to reabsorb the toxins, which can leave us feeling crappy, fatigued or sluggish. It may affect our skin health too. This may or may not surprise you, but there is such a thing as a healthy poo. If you're constipated it may indicate dehydration, a lack of fibre or an imbalanced gut microbiome, but at the other end of the scale if you have diarrhoea, it's not good either and you may be unwell. To give you an idea:

Needs help - e.g. constipated

Ideal healthy poo

Diarrhoea - get this checked out by a GP

To avoid constipation and improve the health of your poo, do as many of the following as you can:

- Make sure you drink two litres of liquids a day (see the hydration section on page 54 for tips).

- Include more soluble fibre in your diet, such as apples, oats, nuts, beans and pulses, whole grains and vegetables.

- Soak chia seeds overnight in a milk of your choice, then add fruits and granola in the morning.

- Do some exercise every day as that stimulates gut motility – the movement helps food to progress along the digestive tract while at the same time ensuring the absorption of the important nutrients.

- If you sit down a lot, get up every 45 minutes.

- Engage in stress-relieving activities, such as deep breathing, stretching and/or meditating.

✷ Summary

The pigments that give fruit and vegetables their bright colours represent a variety of protective compounds. By eating all the colours of the nutrition rainbow, you'll harness their power. However, a healthy digestive system is still fundamental to all aspects of health and if your digestive system isn't working well, it affects your whole body and you might experience bloating, burping or wind. Sitting down to eat, eating slowly and chewing your food thoroughly, ideally around 30 times per mouthful, will all help. Drinking too much water with food dilutes digestive enzymes which may lead to poor digestion and bloating. Avoid drinking too much at meal times, and instead aim to consume water between meals.

Chapter 4

Fats won't make you fat (but they will make you smart)

You may have heard that it's good to eat 'low fat' to help reduce your calorie intake, but 'low fat' foods often have lots of added sugar, salt and artificial additives to make them more palatable.

Real, healthy fats, on the other hand, are a good thing. They can help us feel full up for longer, they help curb our sugar and junk food cravings, and they supply us with essential nutrients that are important for so many aspects of our health, including helping us have moist, plump, glowing skin and nourishing our brains. Examples of what I mean by sources of real, healthy fats are:

- Mixed nuts and seeds, especially chia seeds

- Extra virgin olive oil

- Avocados

- Tofu

- Eggs

- Oily fish

- Full-fat live yoghurt

- Cheese

- Coconut oil

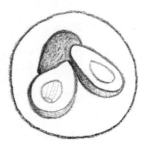

So real, healthy fats are good, but even so fat should make up less than 35% of your daily food intake. In other words, you should eat no more than approximately 70g of fat per day. To give you a sense of what that means, here is the fat content of some popular foods:

- 1 tablespoon of olive oil – 13.5g

- 1 tablespoon of butter – 11g

- Half an avocado – 15g

- 10 almonds – 5g

- 28g Cheddar cheese – 9.3g

ESSENTIAL EGGS – ROCKET FUEL FOR YOUR BRAIN!

Not only does egg yolk contain essential fats, it also contains important fat-soluble nutrients like vitamins A, D and E, and the antioxidants lutein and zeaxanthin. The healthy fats in the egg yolk actually help our bodies to absorb these nutrients too.

What's more, eggs are a great source of something called choline, which is essential for a range of reasons, including creating fats that contribute to strong cell membranes; and producing acetylcholine, an important neurotransmitter that is needed for memory and focus. Eggs are a kind of rocket fuel for your brain!

> ❝ **I wanted to lose weight** *so I cut out all fats from my diet. I chose only low fat or no fat products. After about three weeks my skin was so dry, I had bad dandruff and I felt bad. I also found I was hungrier and didn't lose weight, as I just wanted to eat more of everything else. This carried on for a few more weeks, but then I read about* **how important healthy fats are** *and I now eat avocado, yoghurts, nuts, eggs and oily fish. They keep the skin healthy and stop food cravings as they provide lots of important nutrients and help you feel full up. My skin's all better, I'm now a healthy weight and I do feel full up for much longer than I did when I cut fats out too.* ❞
>
> ## LIVI (15)

Brain health

Did you know that if you take away the water, the dry weight of our brain is made up of 60% fats? These essential fats are called omega-3 fatty acids. We lose some of these fats every day, so unless we replace them through our diet there will be significant changes in our brain function. These fats are critical for normal brain function and development at all stages of our life. In fact, without sufficient vitamins and minerals, our brain's ability to function is affected, creating problems with word recollection, communication, concentration, memory, sleep and so much more.

Fish is in the list above and for good brain health you should aim for three portions of fish a week – ideally two of these should be oily fish – and a handful of mixed, unsalted nuts and seeds daily. The oily fish could be tuna, salmon, mackerel, herring, sardines, trout, kippers or anchovies and it's important because it contains omega-3. As well as promoting healthier brain cells, omega-3 supports neuron growth (basically your brain function) and maintains high levels of the feel-good neurotransmitter dopamine in your brain. Walnuts, chia seeds, flaxseed, pumpkin seeds and (unsurprisingly) omega-3 eggs are also excellent sources of omega-3. If you don't eat fish, you could take algae or fish oil supplements as an alternative.

Nuts are packed with so many nutrients, including lots of vitamins, minerals and essential fats. If you can't eat nuts, seeds have very similar health benefits and can be used in the same way. Here are some ideas for incorporating a handful of mixed nuts or seeds into your daily diet:

- Prepare some trail mix with mixed nuts or seeds and carry it around with you to snack on

- Toss almonds or cashews through a stir-fry

- Add roast chestnuts, pine nuts or seeds to a salad

- Chop any nuts as a crust for fish

- Add nuts or seeds to yoghurt

- Add nuts to home-made cakes or biscuits

- Add chopped nuts to muesli, porridge or a wholegrain breakfast cereal

- Use a nut spread on toast, as a sandwich filling or to fill celery sticks

So there are healthy fats, but there are also unhealthy fats and if we consume too many unhealthy saturated fats, commonly found in fast foods and fried foods, over time they can damage the brain, affecting its ability to process information in particular.

The brain is a very hungry organ. In fact, it uses more energy than any other organ in our body and up to 20% of our nutrient intake goes to fuel the brain. As well as essential fats, it requires proteins, which transport the nutrients to your brain cells, and various vitamins and minerals, particularly iron for brain development, zinc for memory, and vitamins B and D, also key for memory and concentration. It also needs magnesium, flavonoids, found in most fruit and vegetables, and anthocyanins, found in dark berries and other fruit and rich in antioxidants, and choline, from eggs and nuts.

> ❛ **I was having trouble concentrating** at school, so my mum took me to see Tina and she suggested changing my diet to include lots of food to "feed my brain". I started eating a handful of unsalted nuts each day, salmon and mackerel, and lots more fruit and vegetables in things like smoothies and soups. I definitely found that **it helped me focus much more** and I no longer get in so much trouble with the teachers for being fidgety. ❜
>
> ### ROB (15)

Clever carbohydrates

Carbohydrates can be found in lots of different foods and those foods high in complex carbohydrates are important in a healthy diet. However, not all carbs are created equal and some of those foods are healthy, including fruit, vegetables, beans and whole grains, and some are less healthy, such as white bread, white rice and pasta.

The main purpose of carbohydrates – or carbs – in the diet is to provide energy. Most carbs get broken down or transformed into glucose, which can be used as energy.

Dietary carbohydrates provide glucose that body cells can use for energy. In fact, the brain and nerve cells only use glucose for energy. Excess glucose, beyond what the body needs for immediate energy, is converted into and stored as glycogen, but the body can only store enough glycogen to provide about a half-day's supply of energy, so the body must have a frequent supply of complex carbohydrates.

Complex carbohydrates are a good source of fibre. That fibre doesn't provide energy directly, but it does feed the friendly bacteria in your digestive system. These bacteria can use the fibre to produce fatty acids that some of our cells can use as energy, keeping our metabolism healthy and immunity strong.

So which carbs should we be eating? Whole grains (for instance oats, brown rice, whole wheat and quinoa) offer a 'complete package' of health benefits, unlike refined grains (for example white or processed bread, pasta or rice), which are stripped of valuable nutrients in the refining process. Whole grains are packed with nutrients, including protein, fibre, B vitamins, antioxidants (which protect your cells from unstable molecules or free radicals that can cause damage to your cells) and minerals your body needs (iron, zinc, copper and magnesium).

My 16th birthday was coming up *and I seemed to just keep piling on lots of weight, so I thought if I cut out carbohydrates, I would lose a ton of weight. The first thing that happened was that I couldn't sleep, because I was absolutely starving. The next day I was knackered from no sleep and so I ended up craving sugar to give me energy, and ate chocolate bars and drank cans of Coke to keep me going. A nutritionist told me to start eating whole grains, because* **they're broken down more slowly in the body,** *so you don't feel hungry and so they don't cause weight gain like white processed carbs. I now eat things like porridge, granary and seeded bread, brown rice and brown pasta, root vegetables like sweet potatoes, beans and lentils. These foods keep you full up for much longer and so I don't feel like snacking all the time like I did before.*

DERV (19)

SLOW CARBS NEVER NO CARBS!

Complex carbohydrates (such as whole grain bread and brown rice) provide a more stable source of energy as they take longer to digest than simple carbohydrates (like table sugar and syrups). As a source of energy, complex carbohydrates are the better choice.

What's not to love? Carbohydrates fuel your brain, keep you energetic, boost your mood, help you sleep better, improve muscle mass, reduce bloating and aid digestion.

Glorious grains

Many whole grains are naturally rich in an amino acid (a type of molecule that combines to form protein) called tryptophan, which your body needs to produce serotonin, the 'feel-good hormone', and melatonin, the 'sleep hormone'. It therefore follows that eating whole grains, which are high in tryptophan, helps your body establish healthy sleep patterns and has a positive impact on your mental health and overall well-being.

Refined grains that make white flour, white bread, white rice and white pasta are stripped of all the bran, fibre and nutrients, leaving just the starchy carbohydrate. Due to their lack of fibre, white carbohydrates in, for example, pizza, biscuits and many breakfast cereals, can cause major spikes in blood sugar levels, which leads to a subsequent crash that can trigger hunger and cravings for more high-carb foods.

Bran and fibre slow the breakdown of starch into sugars (glucose), thereby maintaining steady blood sugar levels, rather than causing sharp spikes. They help you maintain a healthy weight, whereas refined and processed carbohydrates can drive hunger and make you eat more. That said, it's important not to demonise any foods. Wherever you can, try to choose whole grains to get more nutrients into your diet and improve your energy levels, but cakes, biscuits and pasta are absolutely fine in a balanced healthy diet and can be enjoyed as treats rather than a source of stable energy.

✳ Summary ✳

'Low-fat' foods often have lots of added sugar, salt and other additives to make them taste better. However, real, healthy fats help us feel full for longer, curb cravings and provide many essential nutrients, including omega-3, that support brain function and raise levels of the feel-good neurotransmitter, dopamine. Fish is an excellent source of omega-3 and, if you don't eat fish, you can get omega-3 from algae or fish oil supplements.

Carbohydrates can be divided into 'healthy' and 'unhealthy'. Among the healthy carbs are unrefined (unprocessed) whole grains, which help to produce the happy hormone, serotonin, and the sleep hormone, melatonin. Because they even out hunger-triggering spikes in your blood sugar levels, healthy carbs are good for maintaining a healthy weight and an essential fuel, providing energy for our body and brain. To help you remember: slow carbs NEVER no carbs!

Chapter 5

Balance your blood sugar for all-day energy

Sugar has long been suspected of making some mood and behaviour problems worse. High intakes of sugar and refined starch (from sugary soft drinks, sweets, cakes, biscuits and other ultra-processed foods) rapidly drive up blood glucose levels, unless they are accompanied by enough dietary fibre, fat or protein. The faster your blood glucose levels rise, the more insulin is released and so the faster blood glucose falls again.

The brain's primary fuel is glucose, so it is easy to see how rapid swings in blood sugar could play havoc with mood, behaviour and cognition. In fact, studies have found links between antisocial behaviour and poor blood sugar control.

UP AND DOWN BLOOD SUGAR LEVELS

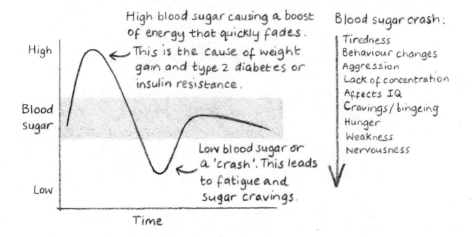

High blood sugar causing a boost of energy that quickly fades. This is the cause of weight gain and type 2 diabetes or insulin resistance.

Blood sugar crash:
Tiredness
Behaviour changes
Aggression
Lack of concentration
Affects IQ
Cravings/bingeing
Hunger
Weakness
Nervousness

Low blood sugar or a 'crash'. This leads to fatigue and sugar cravings.

High / Blood sugar / Low / Time

When your blood sugar levels aren't balanced, it can cause:

- Tiredness
- Lack of concentration
- Lower IQ
- Weakness
- Nervousness
- Behaviour changes
- Cravings/bingeing
- Hunger
- Blood sugar crash
- Feelings of aggression
- Long-term weight gain
- Nausea

TOP TIP

➜ Put a coat on your carbs! By eating, or 'dressing up', your carbohydrates with healthy fats or protein, you slow down their digestion, leading to more stable energy and improved moods throughout the day. ←

Blood sugar

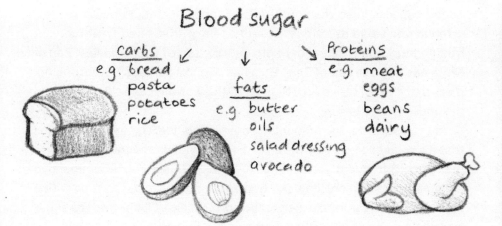

carbs
e.g. bread
pasta
potatoes
rice

fats
e.g. butter
oils
salad dressing
avocado

Proteins
e.g. meat
eggs
beans
dairy

Sugary food and refined white carbs cause the blood sugar to rise and then crash, but there is an answer. The fibre in whole grains, fruit and vegetables cleverly slows down the rate at which the sugars from these foods are digested, giving you much more stable energy and moods throughout the day.

Did you know that we are most likely to binge when our blood sugar is low? This is because low blood sugar makes us hungry and tired, and triggers us to crave foods that will give us a glucose boost as quickly as possible — sugary snacks, bread, pasta, pastries, caffeine or sugary drinks. When you consume these foods, you feel temporary relief and your low blood sugar symptoms disappear, causing you to believe that you're doing the right thing.

Every time these symptoms arise, you reach for the sugar or carbs, your pancreas overshoots to compensate for the blood sugar spike, and your blood sugar dips into the danger zone again. Then the hunger, irritability, anxiety, dizziness and shakiness begin again... and on and on and on it goes.

Added sugar is in so many pre-packed foods, including pasta sauces, ketchup and salad dressings, as well as fizzy drinks and treat foods. A fruit yoghurt and a cereal bar both contain 19g of sugar, while a can of Fanta has 41g and can of Coca Cola has 35g. It's perhaps not surprising, then, that the UK ranks fifth highest in the world for Type 2 diabetes in the under 18 age group.

You can see from the amount of sugar in regular food and drink items that it's so easy to go way over the recommended amounts. I often find that people frequently consume up to four times the recommended amount of sugar in one day. Our bodies are not designed to cope with a high modern sugar intake, hence the current rise of diabetes. The sugar cycle below shows how sugar works on our bodies.

THE SUGAR CYCLE

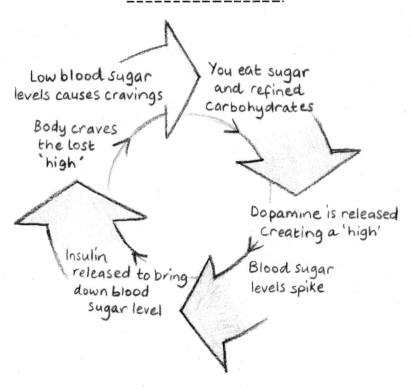

If you don't already have it, download the NHS Food Scanner app and monitor your sugar intake for the next seven days. You may be shocked!

List the five unhealthy foods you find most addictive and have no 'off button' for. Try to consider them as occasional treats rather than everyday foods!

- 1. ....
- 2. ....
- 3. ....
- 4. ....
- 5. ....

MAKING DIETARY CHANGES

Low glycaemic foods have a low value on the glycaemic index. This assigns values to foods based on the effect they have on blood sugar levels two hours later. One of the most effective ways to start dietary changes is to choose low glycaemic foods, which are higher in fibre. Examples are:

- Quinoa, brown rice, amaranth, steel-cut oats, barley, rye, bulgur, wild rice, wheat tortilla, wheat pasta, spelt pasta

- Breads – soya and linseed, wholegrain pumpernickel, heavy mixed grain, whole wheat, sourdough rye, sourdough wheat

- Lentils, chickpeas, kidney beans, black-eyed beans, soya beans

- Asparagus, artichoke, avocado, broccoli, cabbage, cauliflower, celery, cucumber, aubergine, leafy greens, lettuce, mushrooms, peppers, tomatoes, okra, onions, spinach, summer squash, courgette, turnips, beetroot, carrots, sweet potato, corn on the cob

- Oily fish (three times a week)

- Lean meats, white fish, tofu, nuts and seeds

- Garlic, ginger, turmeric

- Non-dairy milks, green tea and plenty of water

SNACK SMARTLY

Snacking can be helpful, but only if it doesn't interfere with proper balanced meals – if you've already filled up on snacks, you may not want to sit down to eat with your family. However, even though you're eating three meals a day, if you get really hungry mid-morning or mid-afternoon you may find snacking tides you over between meal times, but it's important to choose the right snack. Good snack choices – there are some ideas below – can keep your blood sugar levels stable and top up your energy levels, as well as providing a wide range of good nutrients. If you snack and then find you aren't hungry at meal times, though, it's a good idea to quit your snacking.

- Trail mix with seeds, coconut, dried chopped fruit, unsalted mixed nuts and dark chocolate chunks

- Cocoa energy balls

- A smoothie made with green leafy veg, berries and seeds

- Spelt, carrot and walnut muffin

- A hard-boiled egg and two sticks of celery

- Celery sticks filled with no-added-sugar peanut butter

- Half an avocado with an oil and vinegar dressing, and a few toasted pine nuts

- Half an avocado, chopped and mixed with toasted seeds

- Crudités (chopped raw vegetables – try carrots, celery, cucumber and peppers) with a tablespoon of hummus, cream cheese or almond butter

- Six cubes of feta, eight olives and a handful of cherry tomatoes

- Nut butter on apple slices

- Two rye crackers with tinned mackerel in tomato sauce and cucumber

- Two oatcakes with taramasalata, baba ghanoush, smoked salmon or cream cheese, topped with cucumber
- Tuna, celery, cucumber and spring onions mixed with oil and vinegar dressing
- A cup of instant miso soup and a couple of oatcakes
- Hard-boiled eggs on crackers, oatcakes or rye bread
- Beef, salmon or tuna jerky
- Plain or Greek yoghurt with berries, berry compote or stewed apple
- A small cup of berries with a handful of nuts or seeds
- An oatmeal cookie and a piece of fruit
- A slice of seedy banana bread
- Healthy home-made oat or ginger biscuits
- A small handful of Brazil nuts covered in dark chocolate

✳ Summary ✳

Sugary foods and refined white carbohydrates cause blood sugar levels to rise and then crash. **Blood sugar dips can negatively affect your concentration,** attention, focus and IQ, as well as your learning, mood and behaviour. Those blood sugar dips can impact aggression, motivation and even induce hyperactivity. Whole grains, nuts, seeds, pulses, beans, fruit and vegetables contain fibre that slows down the rate at which sugars are digested, **resulting in more stable energy levels.** Too much sugar leaves you hungry and craving more sugar, which could lead to weight gain. It can also cause skin conditions such as acne and tooth decay, and also means you may be at risk of becoming diabetic when you're older, which is why the UK daily recommended amount of sugar is just seven teaspoons.

Chapter 6

Good hydration

You probably know that the human body is mainly water – 72%! But did you know that just a 1–2% drop in your body's optimum water levels can reduce your attention span by 25%? To maximise your concentration and feel at your best you need to stay hydrated, but in order to stay hydrated you need to consume 1.5–2.5 litres of non-caffeinated liquids each day. Keep a bottle near you to sip throughout the day and if you aren't keen on water, pimp it up by adding fresh fruit, cucumber or mint. Remember not to drink too much during mealtimes, as it can affect your digestion.

It's been proved that drinking water slowly throughout the day makes you more hydrated than guzzling lots of water quickly. This makes sense as your intestines can only process so much water at a time and if it goes in too quickly, you'll pee it straight out and lose the benefits.

The common symptoms of dehydration are thirst, dark urine, fatigue, dizziness and headaches, but you can't afford to let yourself become dehydrated, because water does so much for us. For example:

→ To ensure you stay well hydrated, fill and carry a water bottle with you. Add flavour! If you don't like water on its own, add fruit, cucumber or mint. Herbal teas can be a great way to stay hydrated too.

Remember some foods have a high water content so you will be getting water, fibre and nutrients by consuming more of them. These include cucumber, melon, tomatoes, apples, courgettes and aubergines. ←

- It's needed by the brain to manufacture hormones and neurotransmitters (feel-good chemicals)

- It helps form saliva (for digestion)

- It keeps mucous membranes, like your lips or nasal passages, moist

- It helps regulate body temperature, through sweating and respiration

- It allows the body's cells to grow, reproduce and survive

- It acts as a shock absorber for the brain and spinal cord

- It flushes out body waste, mainly via your wee

- It converts the food components needed for survival via the digestion system

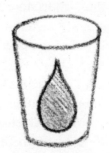

- It lubricates joints

- It helps deliver oxygen all over the body

- It is the major component of most body parts

- It allows the body to absorb and assimilate essential nutrients such as minerals, vitamins, amino acids and glucose

Smoothies

As well as being a way of drinking your liquids, fresh home-made smoothies are a great way to increase your fresh fruit and vegetable intake, and therefore increase your nutrition. It's a fast delivery of vitamins, minerals, enzymes, carbohydrates, chlorophyll (this is the green colour in plants) and countless phytonutrients, which we know can boost health.

A home-made smoothie is in a league of its own compared to an off-the-shelf, processed juice. Some shop-bought juices are stripped of their nutrients through mass production. Others have their natural fructose and fibre removed through pasteurisation or nasty ingredients are added to extend the shelf life, so that carton of juice may not be as healthy as you'd think.

However, juicing fruits removes the insoluble fibre in the flesh and the skin, releasing the sugars. These drinkable fruit sugars are absorbed very quickly into our bloodstream, and that can cause blood sugar spikes and may also damage our teeth. When we consume the whole fruit, the fibre slows down the absorption of the fructose (fruit sugar) and also makes us feel full. Therefore, blending – making smoothies, in other words – is better than juicing as it retains the pulp/fibre and skin of the fruit and veg. The sugar content also means that it's healthier to make fresh smoothies containing more vegetables than fruit. My advice is to make them in the following proportions: 60–80% vegetables to 20–40% fruit.

HEALTH WARNING!

A 1.75l carton of off-the-shelf orange juice may contain the juice of 16 oranges. That juice could have more than three times as much sugar in it as a can of fizzy drink and your body would absorb it in the same way – very quickly – producing an unhealthy sugar boost. So the UK guidelines recommend you consume no more than 150ml a day of any juice due to the sugar content.

Here are some tips for making the healthiest smoothies and juices:

- Aim for rainbow colours – beetroot, carrot, cucumber, tomatoes, watercress, yellow peppers.

- Always include vegetables in the mix and only use a small amount of fruit, such as berries.

- Add some lemon juice or a splash of apple cider vinegar. This will mask the taste of vegetables and make the juice taste sweeter without adding more fruit or sweeteners.

- Including healthy fats, such as chopped walnuts, flaxseeds or nut butter, will slow the absorption of the sugars.

- Tahini provides a boost of calcium.

- Add oats for extra protein.

- Add nut butters for slow-release energy.

The case for avoiding caffeine

Caffeine is the only legal psychoactive drug (that means it acts on the mind) available to under 18s in the UK. Caffeine can have profound stimulating effects on your body. It stimulates the central nervous system (the brain and spinal cord), causing increased alertness and a temporary boost in energy. But it isn't advisable for teenagers to consume caffeine, for many reasons.

It's addictive. Researchers have discovered that even after you stop consuming caffeine, you may experience withdrawal symptoms such as headaches, trouble concentrating and completing tasks, irritability and depression, anxiety, tiredness and sleepiness, and even flu-like symptoms like nausea, muscles aches, and hot and cold spells.

Caffeine may stunt adolescents' development by disrupting the formation of key connections in the brain. During adolescence, when the brain has the most neural connections, caffeine may make the network less efficient.

Caffeine may also cause the body to lose calcium. Consuming too much caffeine could lead to bone loss over time. Drinking coffee, soda or energy drinks instead of milk may also make you more at risk of developing osteoporosis, a condition that weakens your bones when you're older, particularly if you're female. Your teenage years are important for your skeletal growth and development, so you want to avoid anything that might interfere with your calcium levels.

Caffeine takes a major toll on your sleep. Every 10mg of caffeine a 13-year-old boy consumes decreases his chances of getting 8.5 hours of sleep by 12%. Sleep deprivation in adolescents and young people can affect their education, mental health and physical health.

It's true that because caffeine is a stimulant it can help with attention issues and in small doses it can improve headaches, and constipation too, but I recommend that young people do not consume any caffeine at all.

Here are some of the most common sources of caffeine and their caffeine content:

Caffeine source	Caffeine content
Brewed coffee	95–200mg
Coca cola	34mg
Dr Pepper	42mg
Milk chocolate bar	30mg
Peach Snapple	42mg
Mountain Dew	55mg
Iced tea	70mg
Starbucks Frappuccino	115mg
Monster Energy Drink	160mg

Energy drinks are caffeinated (and often very sugary) soft drinks that claim to boost performance and endurance. Consumption of these products has been associated with a number of very serious health complaints if consumed on a regular basis. Teenagers aged between

13 and 17 are among the fastest growing population of caffeine users, with 30–50% of adolescents and young adults being known to consume energy drinks.

Given that energy drink use may cause behavioural problems and negatively impact mental health and well-being (there are numerous studies pointing to this), it is concerning to find that the products are often aggressively marketed at young people like you. In fact, the government is so concerned that as part of its plan to reduce childhood diabetes it intends to ban energy drinks for under 16s.

Up to around one cup of coffee (100mg) a day is considered safe for those that can tolerate caffeine, but if you find you are getting any of the side effects listed above, you may want to cut back, avoid caffeine after midday or swap to decaf.

WHAT ABOUT SPORTS DRINKS?

Sports drinks are often endorsed by celebrities and may be perceived as healthy, because they are often permitted to be sold in schools and at sporting events, so may be consumed in excess.

A study following more than 4100 females and 3400 males for seven years as part of the Growing Up Today Study II found that the more frequently sports beverages were consumed, the greater the likelihood of increased body mass index, leading to both boys and girls becoming overweight or obese.

Sports drinks contain carbohydrate in the form of sugar (glucose or sucrose) or contain no sugar and are flavoured instead with artificial sweeteners. Drinking too many of these, especially when not performing vigorous exercise, can increase the risk of become overweight or obese, and lead to other health problems, such as type 2 diabetes, cardiovascular disease, tooth decay or gum disease.

Alcohol – how it affects us

When we drink alcohol, it's directly absorbed into our bloodstream. From there, it affects our central nervous system, which controls how our body functions, including how we move, see, hear and feel. Under its influence we tend to behave in a completely different manner to the way we would behave if we were sober. In fact, even very moderate amounts of alcohol can make us over-friendly, aggressive or more likely to take risks.

During your teenage years and right up until you are around 25 years of age, your brain is still developing and therefore the teenage brain is much more negatively impacted by alcohol. Binge-drinking can actually kill brain cells in the adolescent brain. It can even cause permanent brain damage in an adolescent.

When you consume a large amount of alcohol in a short space of time (known as binge-drinking), your body can't process the alcohol quickly enough, which can result in alcohol poisoning. Signs include slurred speech, lack of coordination, heavy vomiting and a drop in body temperature – and this is very serious. If you suspect someone has alcohol poisoning, call an ambulance. Don't let the person fall asleep, keep them warm and give them some water. If they do pass out, put them in the recovery position and check their breathing.

HOW CAN I AVOID DRINKING?

Create plans that don't involve drinking alcohol, for example going shopping, to the cinema, a sporting event, a concert or cycling in the park. If you're going to a party, but don't want to drink, plan a strategy in advance, such as taking your own non-alcoholic drinks with you.

Alcohol, sleep and performance

Alcohol depletes the B vitamins vital for mental well-being and energy, and it can be a depressant. It may initially help you fall asleep, but it leads to lighter, diminished sleep and you'll feel very tired the next day. This is because it suppresses melatonin, the sleep hormone, and blocks REM sleep, which is the sleep that really restores your energy levels. Even two or three drinks in one day can create sleep and performance problems for many people, and the more you drink the more it will negatively impact your sleep (for more on why sleep is vital for good health, see page 127).

✳ Summary ✳

For many reasons, it's vital to stay hydrated and that means drinking 1.5–2.5 litres of non-caffeinated liquids each day during your teenage years. Home-made smoothies are a healthy way of increasing your intake of liquids, particularly smoothies, because blending fruit and vegetables retains their fibre, which slows down the absorption of fruit sugars and helps keep our blood sugar levels more balanced. If you're not a fan of water, flavour it with fresh fruit, mint or cucumber.

Although one cup of coffee a day is considered safe, it's much better for your health to avoid caffeine altogether. Try to steer clear of energy drinks, which contain a lot of caffeine, too. Alcohol can be a depressant and can make us feel lethargic, because it depletes the B vitamins that help with energy production. It also negatively influences our sleep quality. Alcohol affects our behaviour and can make us lose our inhibitions, leading us to do things we wouldn't normally do.

Chapter 7

What you eat can make you happier

Many aspects of our lifestyle, such as keeping active, being a non-smoker and maintaining a balanced diet, are important factors in staying physically and mentally healthy. Many studies have demonstrated that a good-quality diet is important and can help with or prevent mental health disorders.

For example, in 2017, all participants in the Australian Smiles Trial were medically diagnosed with moderate to severe depression. After 12 weeks on a predominately plant-based Mediterranean diet rich in colourful fruits and vegetables, fish, legumes, nuts, healthy fats and small amounts of meat, one group showed significantly greater improvements in mental health when compared with another group, which had only received social support. In the dietary support group, 32% of participants achieved full remission, meaning that they were no longer considered depressed. The people who improved their diets the most also reduced their depressive symptoms the most.

DEPRESSION SYMPTOMS

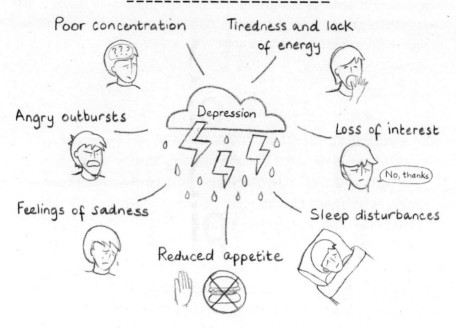

Similarly, also in Australia, the Helfimed Trial (conducted in 2015) showed that a Mediterranean diet can improve mental health in adults suffering from depression – 45% of participants experienced a reduction of depressive symptoms after three months of healthy eating and taking a fish oil supplement.

Fish oil is, of course, a major source of the essential nutrient omega-3 and studies show that lower levels of omega-3 have also been associated with suicidal behaviour and antisocial or aggressive disorders, the latter in both criminal populations and wider society.

In one study, students from Reading University were given 30g of freeze-dried wild blueberries in a flavonoid-rich drink and for a month a positive effect on their mood was observed. Dietary interventions could therefore play a key role in promoting positive mood and perhaps preventing depression.

In fact, there are numerous potential ways in which the quality of your diet may have an impact on your mental health. A poor-quality diet that lacks nutrient-dense foods may make you more susceptible to mental health issues, whereas increasing your dietary intake of folate, zinc and magnesium may reduce depressive disorders and increasing dietary omega-3 fatty acids can reduce anxiety disorders.

> ❝ **I was diagnosed with depression** at 13 and saw a nutritionist who went through my diet. She explained that **what you eat affects how you feel** and she gave me a list of foods to introduce. This included lots of fruit and vegetables, fish, nuts, seeds, lentils, beans and live yoghurt. I made myself daily smoothies with frozen berries and yoghurt too. My thinking patterns were very negative, so I worked on those too, and after a few months I definitely felt much happier in myself. I have read a lot about how **food does help with your mood,** so if you're struggling it's definitely worth a try. ❞
>
> **TESS (17)**

How diet affects our mental health

What we call 'Western' diets – the sort of diets that many people in the UK eat – are associated with higher risk of depression, because they tend to cause low-grade inflammation, when the bacteria in our gut is altered, interacts with our immune system and triggers it in a way that stimulates a response from the body and oxidative stress (see the box on the following page). A healthy Mediterranean diet, on the other hand, reduces inflammation and therefore improves mood, and studies have found that sticking to Mediterranean dietary patterns can reduce inflammation markers.

WHAT IS OXIDATIVE STRESS?

Oxidative stress is a bodily condition that happens when your antioxidant levels are low. It can break down cell tissue and cause cellular damage. This damage can also result in inflammation, which can be linked to depression.

Antioxidants in your body can help protect cells from oxidative stress. They are most abundant in fruits and vegetables (rainbow-coloured foods), as well as other foods, including nuts, whole grains and some meats, poultry and fish.

Here is a list of what you might consume as part of what's usually described as a Mediterranean diet:

- Oily fish, shellfish or algae supplements (vegetarian or vegan)
- Whole grains
- Vegetables, including plenty of leafy green veg
- Fruit, including plenty of dark berries
- Nuts and seeds
- Olive oil and olives
- Green tea
- Herbs and spices
- Water
- Eggs, poultry and dairy
- Dark chocolate

A study conducted by University College London in 2019 showed that people who eat dark chocolate are less likely to be depressed. Chocolate contains a number of psychoactive ingredients (substances that act on the brain), which produce a feeling of euphoria. It also contains magnesium, which is believed to be important for regulating people's moods. Make sure you choose dark chocolate with 70% or more cocoa solids and enjoy a few squares each day. Dark red berries – particularly blueberries, but also blackberries and raspberries – have been shown to improve your memory and mood too. Aim to eat on average a small handful every day.

Having feelings is a normal part of being human and those feelings can be affected by what you eat and drink. However, when you become trapped in an emotional state, for example you can't seem to stop yourself feeling angry or depressed, you may be tempted to turn to food to try to make yourself feel better. That's not a good idea, though, because those food choices can often make you feel worse. So let's just pause for a moment and do a quick check on how you're feeling. Do you identify with any of the emotions in the left-hand column? If you do, read across to the right-hand column for a suggestion on how to look after yourself better.

I feel...	I need to...
Overwhelmed	Take a step back
Stressed	Focus on relaxing
Anxious	Practise coping skills
Sad	Be loving to myself
Angry	Find a positive outlet
Drained	Rest and recharge
Broken	Practise self-compassion
Upset	Take time for myself
Alone	Reach out for support

Get your daily dose of happiness chemicals

Dark chocolate and red berries are simple ways to improve your happiness through what you eat, but there are lots of others. Your brain releases happiness chemicals called neurotransmitters that make you feel good. What you eat actually creates these important messengers, but low levels of them can lead us to feeling low and out of sorts, and imbalanced neurotransmitter production can result in various psychological disorders, so let's look at what you can eat to boost your happiness.

Serotonin – the mood booster

This affects our mood, appetite, learning, memory and sleep. It has been labelled the confidence neurotransmitter, as it boosts our self-esteem and confidence. We make serotonin from an amino acid called tryptophan (amino acids are molecules that combine to form proteins).

Serotonin deficiency can lead to: low self-esteem, being overly sensitive and emotional, anxiety and panic attacks, social phobia, obsessive compulsive disorders, mood swings, depression and insomnia.

Foods that boost serotonin production are: animal products such as turkey, chicken, fish, eggs and cheese; nuts and seeds, for example almonds and sesame seeds; fruit and vegetables, including bananas, kiwi fruit, plums, papaya, dates and tomatoes; and cacao, which is found in dark chocolate.

Dopamine – the motivator

This affects our memory, our learning, and our ability to think and plan. It also helps us strive, focus, find things interesting and get the job done.

Dopamine deficiency can lead to: low self-esteem, lack of motivation or enthusiasm, procrastination, inability to focus, feelings of anxiety and hopelessness, mood swings and fatigue.

Foods that boost dopamine production are: animal products such as turkey, chicken, duck, pork, fish, eggs, cheese, cottage cheese and ricotta cheese; nuts and seeds, for example, almonds, walnuts, sesame and pumpkin seeds; and fruit and vegetables, including bananas and avocados.

GABA – the calming influence

Have you heard of GABA? Like tryptophan, it's an amino acid and it helps us manage stress and control anxiety and fear. It is also important for information processing and improving sleep.

GABA deficiency can lead to: mood disorders, anxiety, depression and insomnia.

Foods that boost GABA production are: animal products such as cow's liver, mackerel and halibut; nuts and seeds, for example almonds, walnuts, soya beans and oats; fruit and vegetables, including bananas, citrus fruits, broccoli and spinach; and fermented and aged foods, such as kimchi (Korean fermented vegetables), sauerkraut (German fermented cabbage) and aged cheese.

Endorphins – the natural high

Have you ever felt a real high after doing some exercise or when you're dancing? Endorphins help reduce stress and anxiety levels, boost our self-esteem, relieve pain and, because they make us feel happy and relaxed, aid sleep. They even help regulate our appetite – when we eat foods that look and taste great, we release endorphins, which help us feel more satisfied by our meals.

Endorphin deficiency can lead to: aches and pains, anxiety, mood swings, impulsive behaviour, depression and insomnia.

Foods that boost endorphin production are: eggs; nuts and seeds, for example unsalted, mixed nuts; fruit and vegetables, such as bananas, citrus fruits, grapes and strawberries; and brown rice, spicy foods (chilli) and dark chocolate.

Tackling mood swings and depression

If you're experiencing mood swings, try upping the quantity of apples, carrots, beans, brown rice and oats you eat. They are all sources of soluble fibre and they work by slowing down how fast the sugar you eat is absorbed into your blood. You don't get as many sugar rushes, which means you don't get as many corresponding sugar crashes, so that's fewer ups and downs.

On the other hand, if you find you feel down a lot of the time, try increasing the whole grains, avocados, walnuts, oily fish and flaxseed in your diet (but make sure the flaxseed is ground, because otherwise your body can't access its nutrients). These are all good sources of essential omega-3 fats. A lack of omega-3 can be associated with depression and so can a lack of folate, which is found in fruit, veg, especially dark, leafy greens, legumes and nuts.

However, it's not just what you eat. Here are some activities that can also help boost our happy chemicals:

Serotonin	Dopamine
• Exercise • Sunshine – get outside every day for at least 10–15 minutes. In winter months, try using a light therapy lamp • Cold showers – blast yourself with cold water for two to three minutes at the end of your daily shower	• Exercise – whichever form of exercise you enjoy the most will give you the biggest increase in dopamine levels • Meditation • Make daily to-do and long-term goal lists – each time you tick off a task or goal, your dopamine levels increase • Do something creative – music, art, crafts, cooking or writing
GABA	**Endorphins**
• Yoga • Meditation • Regular exercise	• Laugh – and cry (ever feel better after a good cry?) • Do something creative – music or art • Exercise • Meditation

The gut and the brain – one system

We have approximately 100 trillion microbes living on us or inside us. We have more of these microbial cells than we do human cells. A couple of kilos of those microbes reside in our gut. It might sound grim, but they play a key role in our health and how we feel.

These microbes are incredibly important to our health and more and more scientific research demonstrates that the microbiome (the name for our gut microbes) affects virtually all aspects of human health, including our immunity, how our body uses nutrients and vitamins, our behaviour and our mental health. The microbiome also affects our brain, because it doesn't operate alone, it's very closely connected to the brain and they work very closely together.

THE GUT/BRAIN CONNECTION

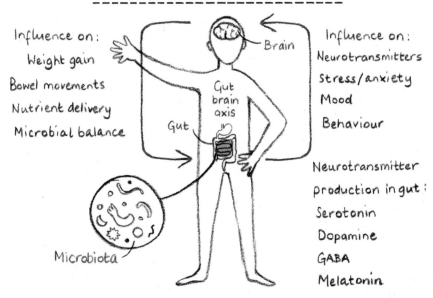

Influence on:
Weight gain
Bowel movements
Nutrient delivery
Microbial balance

Brain
Gut brain axis
Gut
Microbiota

Influence on:
Neurotransmitters
Stress/anxiety
Mood
Behaviour

Neurotransmitter production in gut:
Serotonin
Dopamine
GABA
Melatonin

Your diet directly impacts the health of your gut microbes, so imbalances in microbes can actually inhibit the production of your feel-good hormones. Patients with various psychiatric disorders, including depression, bipolar disorder, schizophrenia and autism spectrum disorder, have been shown to have significant differences in the composition of their gut microbiome.

So what can you do to improve your gut microbiome and mental health? As always, aim to eat a colourful Mediterranean diet rich in plants, fish, legumes, healthy oils and fats, and low in processed and junk foods. Then look to add in foods to feed your microbiome. These are known as probiotic and prebiotic foods, and they will give your gut the fuel it needs for your microbiome to thrive.

Probiotics are live bacteria and although we tend to think of bacteria as causing diseases, probiotic bacteria are actually very good for you, particularly your digestive system, and they help keep your gut healthy. You may notice that they are often added to yoghurts or available as food supplements. Prebiotics, on the other hand, are what probiotics eat. They are a sort of fibre that can't be broken down by the human body and they are present in all sorts of fruit and vegetables.

Probiotics	Prebiotics
Dairy Aged cheeses (Cheddar, Gouda, Parmesan, Swiss) Kefir (a fermented milk made from grains) Live plain or Greek yoghurt	**Fruit** Apples Avocado Bananas (particularly unripe) Kiwi fruit Peaches Pomegranates Tomatoes Watermelon
Fermented foods Kimchi (fermented vegetables) Kombucha (fermented tea) Olives Pickled beetroot Pickles Sauerkraut (fermented cabbage) Soya beans (miso, tempeh)	**Grains and legumes** Barley Porridge oats Rye Wheat Beans (soya, kidney, black, white, including haricot) Chickpeas Lentils

Grains	Vegetables
Sourdough bread	Asparagus
	Cabbage
	Fennel
	Garlic
	Green peas
	Jerusalem artichokes
	Kale
	Leeks
	Mangetout
	Onions
	Savoy cabbage
	Sweetcorn

Other	Nuts
Dark Chocolate (70+% cocoa solids)	Cashews
	Pistachios
	Walnuts

The human brain utilises a whopping 25% of our total energy requirements. Good nutrition is vital so that you can feed your brain the right amount of vitamins, minerals and phytochemicals. Undernourish your brain and poor mental health and behaviours can arise.

Supercharge your immunity

Whether you succumb to viruses often comes down to the state of your body – stress, tiredness and nutrition all play a part. Did you know over 70% of the body's immune cells are located in the gut walls? So good gut health is key to healthy bodily function. As well as ensuring your microbiome is well fed, an antioxidant-rich diet offers huge support for the immune system. Antioxidants play a role in repairing damaged DNA and boosting your body's ability to repair itself, and these antioxidant-rich foods will help support your immunity:

- Apples
- Artichokes
- Berries
- Dark chocolate
- Green tea
- Kidney beans
- Leafy green vegetables
- Oily fish
- Tomatoes

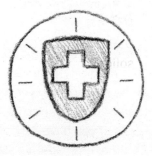

TOP TIP

→ Garlic also contains active ingredients that are anti-bacterial and anti-inflammatory, so enjoy it in lots of your meals. If you start to feel unwell, crush raw garlic and mix it with some olive oil, fresh tomatoes and basil, and eat on a cracker or bread. It works a treat at killing off any potential bugs! ←

Vitamin D

Research shows that having healthy levels of vitamin D, as well as taking a vitamin D supplement, can help keep your immune system healthy and may protect against respiratory illnesses in general. Vitamin D:

- Helps fight colds and flu
- Promotes healthy bones and teeth
- Regulates blood sugar levels
- Plays an important role in regulating mood and warding off depression
- Prevents cancer development
- Reduces the risk of allergies

Some of us are at greater risk of vitamin D deficiency, including people with naturally very dark skin. Larger amounts of the pigment melanin in the epidermal layer result in darker skin and reduce the skin's ability to produce vitamin D from sunlight, resulting in lower vitamin D levels. If you have dark skin – for example, you have an African, African-Caribbean or South Asian background – you should consider taking a daily supplement containing 10 mcg of vitamin D throughout the year.

The NHS recommends that everyone takes a Vitamin D supplement (10 mcg per day) throughout the winter months from September to April. However, while Covid-19 is around they recommend we continue to take it all year round. Vitamin D sprays are also available in any chemist.

Other ways to protect yourself

Stress is known to weaken our immunity, so it's important not to feel overwhelmed and to avoid harbouring negative thoughts. Things like deep-breathing exercises, yoga, meditation and positive affirmations are all really helpful in reducing stress in your body. If you still feel stressed, do speak to an adult and seek a referral to a counsellor or check out the organisation Young Minds.

Regular physical activity helps to boost immune system function by raising levels of infection-fighting white blood cells and antibodies, increasing circulation and decreasing our stress hormones. The key is to try to find an exercise programme that you enjoy. You don't have to be the best at it either – even a 10-minute jog or a long walk will do you the world of good.

Studies have shown that simple handwashing can help prevent a large number of illnesses. Wash your hands before meals or if you've been around others who are sick. And try to avoid touching your eyes, nose and mouth with unwashed hands, as this can provide a virus with a route of entry into your body.

TOP TIP

→ Scientists are also finding more and more health benefits to having a quick blast of cold water in the shower, including boosting your immune system and easing low mood. Experts say the best results come not from a cold shower or bath, but from alternating between hot and cold water. ←

Self-esteem monthly checklist

Confidence isn't about feeling superior to others, it means feeling sure of yourself and your abilities in a realistic, not arrogant, way. Working on our self-esteem should be a regular, ongoing process, and we should all make a point of checking in with ourselves and turning any negative thought patterns ('I can't...) into positive thought patterns ('I can...').

This is a good exercise to do regularly, ideally once a month. Keep a note of your scores so that you can look back and see if there is a direction of travel or pattern. Your self-esteem should improve over time as your nutrition and healthy habits improve.

Rate from 0–10 how much you believe each statement – 0 means you don't believe it at all and 10 means you believe it completely.

RATE YOUR OVERALL SELF-ESTEEM

0   10

I completely dislike who I am   I completely like who I am

What would you need to change in order for you to move up one point on the rating scale? For example, if you rated your self-esteem 6, what would need to happen for you to be a 7?

Statement	Rating
I believe in myself	
I love myself and believe in myself	
I have many good qualities	
I am proud of what I have achieved	
I am excited to try new things	
I accept compliments gracefully	
I learn from my mistakes	
I can cope with criticism	
I focus on success rather than failure	
I am happy with what I see in the mirror	
I am glad I am me – I don't want to be somebody else	
Total score	

✳ Summary ✳

Good mood? Bad mood? Consider your diet and your gut microbes. Studies show that what you eat has an impact on your mental health. A Mediterranean diet that includes lots of fruit and vegetables, as well as oily fish, which contains omega-3, dark berries and dark chocolate, is associated with lower rates of depression. You can also eat to improve the production of the **happiness-boosting neurotransmitters** serotonin, dopamine, endorphins and GABA. Enhancing beneficial bacteria in the gut, for example through the use of probiotic and prebiotic foods, has the potential to improve your mood and reduce anxiety too, and you can improve your immunity through diet as well – garlic, for example, is a potent anti-bacterial and anti-inflammatory.

Chapter 8

Going plant-based

There are various different terms for people who eat a plant-based diet and various different reasons for doing so, including ethical, environmental and nutritional reasons. If you're a vegetarian, you probably only eat fruit and vegetables, grains, legumes, nuts and seeds, but you may eat dairy products (lacto-vegetarian) and eggs (lacto-ovo vegetarian) or fish and seafood (pescatarian) as well. You may even be a vegetarian who very occasionally eats meat or fish (flexitarian) or – at the opposite end of the spectrum – someone who is very strict and not only eats a purely plant-based diet, but also tries to avoid animal-based products such as honey, wool and leather (vegan).

Veganism seems to be becoming more and more popular, and thanks to some amazing advances in food technology it's certainly become much easier to buy what you might call 'vegan convenience food'. However, some of these new products may be vegan, but they are still what are called ultra-processed foods and may contain lots of extra sugar or saturated fats, or additives to thicken or to add colour and texture. Eating more plants and less meat is generally considered to be good for your overall health, but if you're simply swapping meat for non-meat ultra-processed foods then your health is unlikely to benefit, with obesity, type 2 diabetes, heart disease and cancer being some of the possible outcomes. Make sure you read the labels, so you know what you're consuming, and try to eat as much genuinely plant-based food as you can.

Did you know that some vitamins and minerals can be stored by the body for up to a year? This means that when you first become a vegan you may feel great, but over time the lack of essential nutrients can have a serious effect on your health. Some people become vegans without doing any research. However, most types of meat and fish are good sources of essential nutrients, so simply cutting out whole food groups without planning how you're going to replace those nutrients isn't ideal.

Being a healthy vegan

In fact, eating an 80% plant-based diet is safe and very healthy. However, consuming no animal products at all may create health issues and there are ten key nutrients that can be lacking in a vegan diet.

Calcium

Dairy – milk and cheese – is a primary source of calcium for non-vegans and calcium is important for strong, healthy bones, but it also has a role in regulating muscle contractions, so it helps to control the beating of your heart. Good vegan sources of calcium include oranges, red kidney beans, chickpeas, tahini, kale and cavolo nero. Also, take a look at the label on your alternative milk and make sure it's fortified with calcium. Most are, and many contain added vitamin D and B12 too.

Vitamin A

If you've been feeling less than 100%, it could be because you're lacking vitamin A, which boosts your immune system and makes your skin glow. For most people, the main sources are eggs, yoghurt and oily fish, but unfortunately vegans don't eat any of those. Luckily, the body can convert the beta-carotene found in red vegetables (peppers), orange vegetables (carrots and sweet potatoes) and yellow fruits (apricots, mangoes and papayas) into vitamin A.

Iron

Iron is essential for the production of red blood cells, but if you don't get enough of it you may become anaemic, causing you to feel incredibly tired. There are two forms of iron, but the form found in plants is much harder for the body to absorb, so you should include at least one plant-based source of iron in every meal. That means fortified breakfast cereals, dried fruit, nuts, seeds, dark green leafy veg, tofu, tempeh, beans, pulses and lentils. In fact, try basing each meal around BLT – not bacon, lettuce and tomato, but beans, legumes and tofu – and add onion and garlic, as they have been shown to make iron (and zinc) more available to the body. Vitamin C, found in fruit, fruit juices, broccoli and red peppers, can also help improve the absorption of iron and tea can hinder it.

Vitamin B12

Vitamin B12 keeps nerve and blood cells healthy. You only need 2.4mcg of it a day, but vegans often don't get enough of it and, although you may not realise a lack of it is the cause, it could be why you feel tired, weak or even depressed. The only reliable vegan sources of B12 are fortified foods such as plant milks, some soya products and breakfast cereals, but even these probably won't provide sufficient B12, which is why I recommend you consider vitamin B12 supplements.

Omega-3

Omega-3 helps reduce inflammation in your body and it's often referred to as 'essential' because it can only be obtained through your diet. Plant sources such as quinoa, dark green leafy vegetables, nuts, seeds and seed oils are useful, but because the body has to do some conversion work to access the omega-3, I recommend you think about a vegan omega-3 supplement derived from algae oil (oily fish are such a great source of omega-3 for fish-eaters because algae is a great source of omega-3 and fish eat a lot of algae!).

Zinc

The best sources of zinc are dairy, meat and shellfish, none of which are options for vegans, but plant sources are plentiful and include avocados, dark green leafy vegetables, tofu, lentils, oats, sourdough bread and seeds.

Choline

Choline isn't a particularly well-known nutrient, but it's important for brain health. Small quantities of it can be made by the liver, but not enough for all the body's needs, so it's vital to include sources in your diet. Vegetables such as broccoli, kale and cavolo nero are all good sources of choline.

TOP TIP

→ **Vegans and vegetarians need to consume 1.8 times more iron than omnivores! That's because there are two forms of iron and the human body finds it harder to absorb the one found in plant-based foods (this is known as non-haem iron, whereas the one found only in animal products is haem iron). Always think to include BLT – beans, legumes or tofu – at mealtimes.** ←

Iodine

Our bodies require iodine to grow and to maintain a healthy metabolism and normal thyroid function. Whole grains, green beans, courgettes, kale and strawberries are plant sources of iodine, but levels depend on how much iodine there was in the soil in which the plants were grown and can be low. For vegans, seaweed is a good source, but as you can have too much iodine, have it just once a week. Alternatively, I recommend a daily multivitamin or a sea kelp or spirulina supplement.

Vitamin D

Known as the sunshine vitamin, because your body makes it when your skin is exposed to sunlight, many people can be deficient in it during the winter, when natural light is in short supply, and those with darker skin can be deficient in it all year round. This matters because vitamin D is essential for boosting your immune system, maintaining muscle strength and reducing the risk of depression. Ideally you need at least 10mcg daily, and mushrooms and fortified foods like plant milks are reliable sources, but I recommend taking a supplement from September to April, and all year round if you have darker skin.

Protein

If you're following a vegan diet, it's important to eat a wide range of proteins to ensure you're taking in all the essential amino acids, because many plant-based foods deliver some but not all of them. Those that do include tofu, tempeh, edamame beans, quinoa, buckwheat (found in soba noodles), beans, legumes, seitan, nutritional yeast, nuts and nut butters, amaranth, hemp seeds and chia seeds, and vegan Quorn products.

How to get the nutrients you need as a vegan

As the healthy vegan plate illustration shows, if you're a vegan you should aim to fill half your plate with vegetables and fruits, a quarter with grains and starches, and a quarter with plant-based proteins. Balancing every plate with plant proteins is key – jackfruit, for instance, doesn't contain any protein! Include wholefood fats, such as avocado and olive oil, and fortified plant-based dairy, such as oat milk, in the meal, on the side or as a snack, but bear in mind that supplements may be needed.

You require more nutrients in your teens than you do at any other time of your life, so, as I've said, I recommend vegans should ideally take vitamin B12, vitamin D and iodine (multivitamin) supplements, and the Vegan Society is an inexpensive place to buy these from. In fact, the Vegan Society produces a range of supplements, including Veg 1, which is a chewable tablet containing key nutrients, although not calcium or omega-3 (the first ingredient on the list is sugar, but this is to help with the taste as it's chewable).

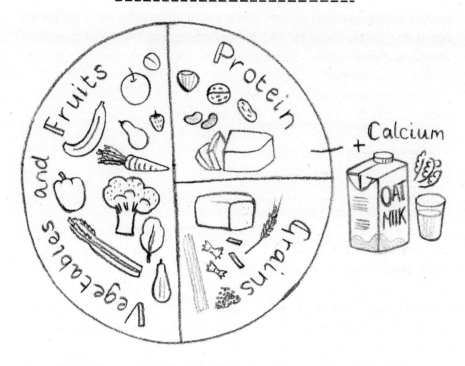

There are also other companies that produce excellent-quality vegan supplements, including Cytoplan and Wild Nutrition. In comparison to many products on the market, these contain no unnecessary preservatives, colourants, fillers or binding agents. They are also free from aggressive doses of synthetic or isolated ingredients often found in traditional, compressed powder tablets, which often pass through the body, unable to be used. Not only are food state nutrients better absorbed by the body, they're kinder to the digestive system too.

Protein-combining

As mentioned above, vegans and vegetarians should try to combine different sources of protein in the same meal. To explain why this is, I need to talk about the building blocks of protein, which are called amino acids (AAs). There are nine essential AAs and 11 non-essential AAs. Non-essential AAs can be made in the body, but essential AAs must be obtained from food sources. However, few plant sources can provide all nine essential AAs in one go – examples of incomplete proteins like this include beans, grains, rice and nuts – so you need to mix it up to get the full range. Some ideas for vegetarian meals and snacks that contain complementary proteins include:

- Yoghurt with nuts and muesli
- Peanut butter on whole grain toast
- Whole grain pitta and hummus
- Macaroni and cheese
- Beans with tortillas or tacos and rice
- Broccoli, cheese and pasta bake
- Lentil or bean soup with pasta
- Granary or rye bread and cheese sandwich
- Tofu with any grain e.g. rice, quinoa, barley or buckwheat

For vegans, the reasons and the principles for protein-combining are the same, but obviously vegans don't eat dairy, so the ideas are slightly different:

- Bean soup and crackers
- Black beans and rice
- Pasta and peas
- Wholewheat bread and peanut butter
- Wholegrain pitta bread and hummus
- Spinach salad topped with nuts and seeds
- Lentil soup with wholegrain bread
- Barley and lentil soup
- Noodles and peanut sauce
- Spinach and chickpea curry

DAILY FOOD REQUIREMENTS FOR VEGANS

Food group	Suggested daily intake
Fruit and vegetables: fresh, frozen, dried or tinned, including all the colours (white, yellow, orange, red, purple and green)	At least 5 x 80g (fist-sized) portions; 1 x 30g if one of the five is a portion of dried fruit
Leafy greens: including cabbage, kale, spinach, broccoli, pak choi, watercress and rocket	2–3 x 85g portions
Starchy foods: including oats, sweet potatoes, wholemeal bread, wholewheat pasta and brown rice	5 x 30g (fist-sized) portions, preferably all whole grains
Protein-rich foods: including tofu. soya milk, soya yoghurt, beans, chickpeas, lentils and peanuts	2–3 (palm-sized) portions
Healthy fats: including nuts, seeds, avocado, olives, olive oil, coconut or nut yoghurt (all rich in omega-3)	1 x 30g (palm-sized) portion of nuts or seeds or ½ an avocado (for more on quantities see page 31)
Calcium-rich foods: including calcium-fortified plant milks, calcium-set tofu or other calcium-fortified foods	400ml of calcium-fortified plant milk is two-thirds, or 100g (raw weight) of calcium-set tofu is half, of the recommended daily intake for adults

By incorporating more plant-based meals into your diet, you will not only save money, but you will also be helping our environment. Even if you're not vegetarian or vegan, aim to eat exclusively plant-based meals at least one day a week, if you can.

If you do eat meat and fish, look out for the 'Farm-assured Food Standards Red Tractor', the 'RSPCA monitored' and the 'ASC Farmed Responsibly' signs on supermarket food in the UK.

I know I've always been a picky eater *and I've never really liked meat. When I went completely plant-based, I ate a lot of toast, pasta, pizza, pasties and vegan sausages, and I admit I didn't have a lot of fresh food. After a few months of that I didn't feel great. I had dark circles under my eyes and my skin really got me down – I had a combination of oily T-zone and spots, and then dry patches like eczema over my body. I was tired all the time and really troubled by insomnia – I found it difficult to get to sleep and then I woke up early. I was also more generally anxious and I didn't feel motivated at school. The thing was,* **I didn't realise that my diet was far too narrow** *to give me all the nutrients I needed to support my mental and physical health. Once I made myself not be so fussy and varied my diet a bit, and started taking regular supplements to make sure I got all the important nutrients, I felt ten times better in just a couple of weeks.*

ISLA (14)

✳ Summary ✳

It's true there are significant health benefits to a plant-based diet, not only for us, but also for our planet. However, there is a risk that you will lack some essential nutrients, so ensure you get all the nutrients you need by **understanding what you need to include in your diet** every day and planning your menus. By taking a vegan multi-nutrient formula and algae omega-3 supplement you can also protect yourself from any potential nutrient deficiencies, and bear in mind that going 80% plant-based is not only safe and healthy, but also, from a nutritional point of view, easier to achieve than going exclusively vegan.

Chapter 9

Love the skin you're in

Your skin is a reflection of what's going on inside your body. Poor skin can indicate that something is amiss internally. In our teenage years, we require a huge amount of nutrients – more than at any other time in our lives. The food choices you make can either boost or diminish your skin's glow. For you to really have clear, healthy skin, you need to ensure that your diet is rich in some key nutrients, such as zinc, vitamin A, vitamin C and essential fats, as well as keeping hydrated and ensuring you do a poo every day to remove toxins from your body.

Every 35 days, our epidermis (the outer layer of our skin) uses the nutrients we eat (the building blocks of our cells) to replace itself, so your food has the power to nourish or harm your complexion. Whenever imbalances arise, and our skin doesn't look as healthy as we'd like it to, they are likely due to a combination of factors. These can include stress, hormonal issues, poor diet and water intake, prolonged lack of sleep, digestive or liver issues, lymph circulation, toxins and even cigarette smoke.

The reason I became a nutritionist is because I had severe acne from the age of 14 and I discovered, after several years of suffering, that what I ate made a <u>huge difference</u> to my skin.

We also know that stress and acne influence each other, so the psychological aspect of acne is not to be underestimated, as negative stress can make the skin more susceptible to inflammation and, therefore, pimples. Exercise, on the other hand, naturally reduces the levels of stress hormones in the body and that's good for your skin.

There is a wealth of research now that shows how important it is for us to maintain good gut health in order to have healthy skin. Put simply, our gut microbiome is a vast collection of bacteria, viruses and fungi that influences the immune system, helps produce certain nutrients and can control inflammation in the rest of the body.

An overabundance of mainly bad bacteria can disrupt the role of the gut in digestion and absorption, and lead to inflammation through the by-products from bad bacteria and by stopping the body utilising the essential nutrients we need for skin health. To love our skin we also need to love our gut bacteria, which is why we recommend feeding our microbiome the foods it loves (see pages 71–72).

Diet and skin health

Recent studies have looked at a number of skin conditions, such as acne, eczema, ageing skin and psoriasis, in conjunction with diet. Certain nutrients, foods or dietary patterns may act as triggers for inflammation in the skin, or they may actively reduce inflammation and energise skin at a cellular level.

In terms of beneficial effects, an eating pattern that emphasises the consumption of whole foods over highly processed foods is the golden rule. So eating a rainbow diet (see page 25), whether you are vegan, pescatarian, flexitarian or omnivore, is the basis for getting all the right micronutrients and phytonutrients we need for healthy skin – but we also have to think about our intake of sugar and fats.

Sugary foods

Sugar and refined carbohydrates are linked to inflammation in the body and sugary foods affect our blood glucose levels (see page 47), which can create havoc for the skin. Sugary foods are fine in moderation, but try to swap some of the refined, white carbs – cakes, crisps, white bread, white rice – for whole grains to help improve your skin.

Fatty foods

It is good to recognise that there are healthy fats and unhealthy fats, which can affect the condition of our skin. Omega-3 is one of the healthy ones. It can improve the texture of dry skin, reduce the severity of acne, reduce inflammation underneath the skin's surface, assist with the healing process and even slow down the ageing process. Researchers have also found that a diet high in omega-3 can make the skin less reactive to UV rays, which is good news for reducing skin damage. Studies show that 87% of UK teenagers consume insufficient omega-3 in their diet. Food sources include oily fish, especially cold-water fatty fish such as salmon, sardines and herring, walnuts, flaxseeds and chia seeds. Monounsaturated fats are also healthy and play an important role in keeping skin soft and supple. Food sources of these include avocados, olives and extra virgin olive oil.

TOP TIP

→ Sugar and refined carbohydrates are linked to inflammation in the body and sugary foods affect our blood glucose levels (see page 47), which can create havoc for the skin. Try making your own sweet treats with fruit such as bananas, frozen berries and dates rather than consuming too many ultra-processed sugary snacks like biscuits, cakes and sweets. ←

How to have healthy skin

- Drink at least two litres of filtered water each day (this can be in herbal teas too)

- Avoid sugary drinks and caffeine, and drink herbal and decaffeinated green tea instead

- If eliminating cow's milk for a month helps, swap your regular milk for nut, oat, coconut or rice milk

- Drink a green smoothie as often as you can

- Follow a nutrient-dense, whole food, diverse diet with minimal intake of nutrient-poor processed and junk foods

- Eat something from each colour of the rainbow every day or even at every meal

- Eat plenty of fish and shellfish for their omega-3 and anti-inflammatory benefits

- A diet high in anti-inflammatories and rich in beta-carotene, which converts to vitamin A, is helpful, so eat carrots, sweet potato, squash, broccoli, spinach and kale

- Eat healthy fats, such as avocados, walnuts, flaxseeds, nuts and seeds

- Have plenty of leafy green vegetables every day, not just broccoli, spinach and kale, but also vegetables with dark green leaves, such as watercress, chard and pak choi

- Aim to consume lots of nutrient-rich whole grains such as oats, quinoa and black rice, and legumes, such as lentils and beans – these have lots of fibre, which feed your gut bacteria

- Opt for lean, white meat, rather than red meat, like beef and lamb, which can be fattier

- Eat dark berries, as they are a potent anti-inflammatory

- Use as many herbs – dried or fresh – as you can to increase your healthy gut bacteria

- Cut down or cut out fried foods, such as chips or fast food, as they may promote inflammation

- Avoid foods high in refined sugars, artificial preservatives, additives, colours and other chemicals that are often added to processed foods

LIFESTYLE HABITS THAT IMPROVE SKIN HEALTH

- Exercise increases blood flow and provides more oxygen to our skin

- Exercise reduces stress-related acne

- Exercise 'cleans' the body – sweating has a positive effect because your pores open up and excess sebum and dirt are removed naturally

- Wash your skin with a gentle cleanser or water after you exercise to ensure you wash away all the toxins you release

- Meditation and breathing exercises can also help reduce stress

How to treat acne

Acne is one of the most common dermatological conditions, affecting millions of young people and adults worldwide, although the triggers for acne can change according to your life stage. Hormones are commonly blamed for acne, but diet affects hormones, so it makes sense to do the groundwork on your diet rather than trying to treat acne using medication as the first step.

Dairy, specifically milk, has been linked to acne. It can cause a reaction that produces sebum, potentially causing an overproduction of oil, followed by blocked pores and acne. Be aware that whey and casein protein powders can create the same response.

If you want to see whether dairy is creating an issue for your skin, try cutting out all dairy, including milk, cheese and yoghurt, for a month. During this period, monitor your skin – for example, you could take before and after pictures. You may find that hard cheeses and live natural yoghurts don't cause a problem for you, so try to reintroduce those as soon as you can as they are a great source of calcium.

If you're cutting out dairy products, it's important to replace them with calcium-rich foods, including canned fish such as sardines or salmon with bones, beans and lentils, soya beans and soya products such as calcium-set tofu soya yoghurt or tempeh, seeds, tahini, almonds, dried figs, certain leafy greens like kale, pak choi, and collard and turnip greens, and calcium-fortified cereals, breads and milks.

In one study, acne sufferers on a 10-week low sugar diet saw a significant improvement in the appearance of their acne, plus decreased inflammation and lower stress hormones, so it is possible to make improvements in a fairly short period, but commitment to dietary changes is key!

TOP TIP

→ Smoothies are great when you want a speedy, nutrient-dense breakfast option and an easy way to incorporate more nutritious vegetables into your diet – try my recipe for tasty green smoothie (see page 210). ←

How to treat eczema

Dry, itchy skin is no fun, as those who suffer from eczema know all too well. It often develops as a result of inflammation in the body, so eating foods that do not cause inflammation may help reduce symptoms. An anti-eczema diet is, in fact, very similar to an anti-inflammatory diet and so is great for better gut health and energy. Focus on the following:

- Foods high in inflammation-fighting flavonoids and vitamin C, such as colourful fruits like cherries and leafy green vegetables, especially kale and broccoli

- Lean chicken and turkey, and white fish, salmon, mackerel and sardines

- Vitamin E-rich foods, such as almonds, pine nuts, sunflower seeds, avocado, avocado oil and dried apricots

- Lentils, chickpeas, kidney beans, black-eyed beans and soya beans

- Soya and linseed bread, wholegrain pumpernickel, heavy mixed grain, whole wheat, sourdough rye and sourdough wheat (this is fine as long as gluten is not a trigger)

- Non-dairy milks

- Foods that are high in zinc, such as seafood, lean red meat, pumpkin seeds and dark chocolate

✳ Summary ✳

For healthy, glowing skin you need to follow a healthy, nutrient-rich diet and have a positive lifestyle. Where possible, try to manage stress levels through healthy lifestyle practices like daily exercise, relaxing breathing techniques, yoga, meditation or simply enjoying time in nature and chatting with friends and family. Using topical creams to tackle issues externally as well as internally may also be appropriate. However, for some of us it can take a while before we see the results of any changes we make, but don't be hard on yourself. Take it step by step, enjoy the journey – and your skin will improve in time.

Chapter 10

Achieve a healthy weight for life

Imagine a life where you feel fantastic every day, full of energy and vitality, you have stable moods, a positive mindset and are fully content with and confident about your body. My goal is for you to accept a healthy, realistic weight for yourself and to love your body just the way it is, not be constantly striving to be an unhealthy, 'thin' version of yourself.

Diets don't work

I've worked with thousands of teenagers and adults whose daily quest is to be thin and stay thin. They develop rigid behaviours and thinking patterns, and can't relax and enjoy their daily lives because they are consumed with worrying about weight gain. This is tragic, and many of them express extreme sadness at how limiting these behaviours and thoughts are to their achieving happiness and a sense of well-being.

They may constantly restrict food, skip meals, avoid social occasions, go on fad diets or spend days feeling hungry to try to keep their weight down. The consequences of this could be an inability to concentrate, mood swings, poor skin, poor sleep and exhaustion, all due to a lack of the important nutrients that we need to thrive. In the long term, it can lead to a number of health issues, such as poor bone health and hair loss, and can even impact upon the ability to have children.

A healthy weight is achieved by nourishing your body with all the important food groups and, what's more, eating nourishes our soul as well as our bodies. Sitting around the table to eat a meal is an essential bonding ritual for families and with friends. Diets often mean that you can't join in with so many of life's joyful activities, leaving you feeling isolated and missing important social occasions and events. Here are some of the downsides of diets:

- Dieting impairs your thinking, memory and mood
- Extreme dieting can damage the kidneys, heart, immune system and brain
- Dieting reduces bone mass – 45% of skeletal mass develops in teenage years and stays with you for the rest of your life, so it's important to feed your bones during this vital growth period

If you're concerned about your weight, it's important to avoid all faddy diets that cut out important food groups like fats and carbohydrates. These food groups are so important for fuelling your body and provide lots of important nutrients that make you feel happy and energised. Let's look at some basic guidelines on how to achieve a healthy weight for the rest of your life, not just your teenage years.

Ditch the scales – most of us will fluctuate in weight each day depending on our daily food intake, drinks, hormone changes, exercise and activity levels and even sleep. Constantly weighing yourself is an unhelpful activity that can lead to compulsive behaviours and anxiety.

There is a big difference between a 'healthy weight' and a 'cosmetically desirable weight'.

Cut back on sweetened drinks

Perhaps one of the easiest ways to maintain a healthy weight is to cut back on sweetened beverages. Fizzy drinks, energy drinks, shop-bought fruit drinks, fruit juices and sweet teas are loaded with added sugars or just simply a huge quantity of natural sugar from the juice of fruits. When we eat a piece of fruit, we consume the fibre, which slows down the rate of absorption of the sugars. Whole fruit is super-healthy, but fruit juices mean we can consume large amounts of sugars in one hit, which can lead to a blood sugar dip (see page 47).

Studies show that high added sugar consumption can lead to weight gain in teenagers and may also increase their risk of certain health conditions, such as acne, type 2 diabetes and non-alcoholic fatty liver disease, as well as tooth decay. Research also indicates that teenagers are more likely to consume sugary beverages if their parents do, so it's beneficial to cut back on these unhealthy drinks as a family.

Fuel your body with nourishing foods

Rather than focusing on calorie content, choose foods based on the amount of nutrients, including vitamins, minerals and fibre, that they contain. Because as teenagers you are still growing, you have higher needs for certain nutrients – such as iron, phosphorus and calcium – than adults. The Aggregate Nutrient Density Index (ANDI) is a scoring system that rates foods based on their nutrient content and you might be interested to know that the most nutrient-rich foods on the planet are: all green leafy vegetables, salmon, liver, blueberries, pulses, eggs, garlic, shellfish and oats.

Vegetables, fruits, whole grains, healthy fats, and wholesome protein sources are not only nutritious, but may also encourage the maintenance of a healthy weight. For example, the fibre found in vegetables, whole grains and fruits, as well as the protein found in sources like eggs, chicken, beans and nuts, can help keep you full between meals and may prevent overeating by keeping blood sugar levels stable.

Don't avoid fat

Because your bodies are still developing, teenagers need to eat more fat than adults. When trying to lose weight, some people think it's a good idea to cut out sources of dietary fat due to their calorie content. However, cutting out fats can negatively impact growth, mental health and proper brain development (your brain continues to develop until you're about 25 years old).

Instead, focus on swapping unhealthy fat sources for healthy ones. Replacing unhealthy fats, such as deep-fried foods, cakes and ice cream, with nuts, seeds, avocados, olive oil and fatty fish can promote healthy weight loss. The fact is, good fats keep us feeling full up for longer and stop sugar cravings too. Head back to Chapter 4 for more on the benefits of healthy fats.

Limit added sugars

It's not uncommon for teenagers to love eating foods high in added sugars, such as sweets, biscuits, sugary cereals and other sweetened, processed foods. But if you're trying to focus on your health and a positive body weight, cutting back on added sugars is essential.

This is because most foods that are high in added sugars are low in protein and fibre, which can cause your appetite to fluctuate and may lead to overeating throughout the day. The blood sugar dips that come after eating high-sugar foods can make you feel even more hungry! Rather than snacking on these foods, why not try more savoury snacks (see pages 52–53 and the recipe section, which starts on page 175).

Avoid fad diets

A study in 16 young women found that those who drank a high-sugar beverage in the morning reported greater feelings of hunger and consumed more food at lunch than those who consumed a lower-sugar breakfast drink. High-sugar foods not only drive hunger, but may negatively impact mood, academic performance and sleep in teenagers.

The pressure to lose weight quickly can cause teenagers to want to try fad dieting. There are countless fad diets, some promoted by popular celebrities and influencers. It's important to understand that diets, especially restrictive fad diets, never work long term and can even be harmful to health.

Overly restrictive diets are so hard to stick to and can't deliver all of the nutrients your body needs to function at an optimal level. What's more, eating too few calories can slow weight loss as your body adapts in response to limited food intake.

Instead of focusing on short-term weight loss, you should concentrate on achieving slow, consistent, healthy weight loss over time. Balance your plate (50% fruit and vegetables, 25% protein and 25% whole grains – see page 32) and take on board all the advice in this section.

Eat your veggies

Vegetables are packed with fibre and water, which can help you feel full and more satisfied after meals. This decreases the chance of overeating by keeping your appetite stable throughout the day. They also feed the microbiome (gut bacteria), which is important for our metabolism, so by feeding the gut bacteria what it needs to thrive, you will enjoy improved metabolism. Aside from being highly nutritious, research has shown that consuming veggies can help teenagers reach and maintain a healthy body weight.

Add in physical activity

If you want to improve your physical fitness, there are various ways to go about it and you don't have to join a gym, start running or take up a sport (not that these aren't good things to do, because they are). To begin, what you have to do is just move more and sit less.

If you improve your daily activity levels, you may discover you lose weight naturally. You could also increase your muscle mass and that can help your body burn calories more effectively. Experiment! There are so many new activities or sports to try, so keep going until you find something you really enjoy.

Set healthy, realistic goals

Losing excess body fat can be a good way to get healthy. However, it's important to have realistic weight and body image goals. If you're overweight, I completely understand that losing excess body fat will be important to you, but the focus should always be on improving health, not just body weight.

Having a realistic weight goal can be helpful for some people. However, improving your diet and increasing physical activity can be much more effective overall. It's so important to understand that everyone has a different body shape and type, and, although you may desire to be a particular body shape, this may not be achievable for you unless you become extremely unwell. Learning to love our bodies for all the amazing things they do for us is the first step to self-acceptance and self-love. Once we start nourishing and nurturing our bodies through healthy lifestyle habits, improved dietary choices and enjoying exercise that suits us, I find everyone starts to feel happier and more confident with both their bodies and themselves.

✳ Summary ✳

Diets don't work. They are unsustainable, and a healthy weight is achieved by nourishing your body with all the important food groups. Eating a natural diet with more plant-based foods, and plenty of fibre, healthy fats and protein with each meal, will ensure you don't get blood sugar dips, which drive hunger and sugar cravings. Be aware of the bliss point, where foods, particularly ultra-processed and takeaway foods, are produced with exactly the mix of salt, sugar and high fat to create food cravings and be addictive, and if you want to enjoy sweet treats eat them with main meals as a dessert, ensuring you don't get blood sugar spikes, because the rest of the meal will be digested slowly.

Chapter 11

Gain weight and bulk up healthily

It's not particularly healthy to be overweight, but at the same time it's not particularly healthy to be underweight either, especially if it's because there are issues with your nutrition. However, here are some healthy ways to put on weight:

- **Eat more often.** If you tend to feel full quite quickly, rather than three big meals, have five or six smaller ones throughout the day.
- **Snack attack.** A little and often may be the key for you, as long as your snacks are healthy ones, like nuts, seeds, dried fruit or a small piece of cheese.
- **Choose whole grains**. These are rich in nutrients, and wholegrain breads and cereals, when combined with lean protein, fruit and veg and dairy products, will all help you gain weight.
- **Calorie-boosters.** Add grains, rice or root veg to soup, add some grated cheese or avocado to baked beans or scrambled eggs – find healthy but almost unnoticeable ways to increase the calorie count of your meals.

- **Drink up**. If you drink before or during a meal, you may find it stops you feeling really hungry. Instead, try small sips with your food or don't drink until half an hour after you've eaten.

- **Be treat-wise.** A big piece of cake makes a nice treat and would certainly contribute towards weight gain, but it also contains a lot of sugar and fat. If you can, stick to healthier treats like muesli bars or whole grain biscuits or treats like home-made muffins. (head to page 211 for some inspiration).

- **Keep fit.** Exercise can help you put on weight by building muscle and it may make you feel hungrier too.

The best weight-gain foods

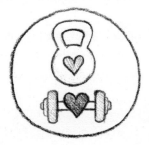

Protein is an important part of your weight-gain diet, but there's a point after which more protein isn't necessarily better – it's just more (this is due to a process called protein synthesis, which means there's only a certain amount of protein your muscles can absorb in one sitting). The ideal quantity of protein for all of us is around 20–30% of our overall diet. The best plan is to space your protein out in 20–40g doses throughout the day. Good sources of protein are:

- Lean meat – beef, lamb, pork
- Poultry – chicken, turkey, duck
- Fish and seafood
- Dairy products – milk, yoghurt, cheese
- Plant proteins – beans, lentils, legumes, soya, tofu, nuts, seeds and whole grains

Fats are a vital part of your diet, because they promote brain and hormone function, and help your body make the most of certain vitamins. Fats also contain roughly double the calories per gram of protein and carbohydrates (about 10 calories per gram versus about five calories per gram). Foods with a high fat content usually taste pretty good, too, so you would be forgiven for thinking that piling on the fatty foods is an easy way to pile on the pounds, but it's not as simple as that.

What you need to do is ditch the doughnuts and steer clear of the unhealthy fats, and concentrate on the healthy fats, like nuts and seeds, avocados, olive oil and oily fish, because they will help with weight gain, while benefiting your overall health.

Compared to protein and carbs, fats also have a much lower 'thermic effect'. That means your body burns anywhere from 5 to 30% fewer calories digesting fats than it does the other two macronutrients. The fewer calories your body expends to digest the food, the more weight you can retain.

An easy way to up your diet's fat content is to cook your meat and vegetables in olive, coconut or another calorie-rich oil. Aim to add in these healthy fats wherever you can to increase your weight:

- Full-fat milk, butter, cheese and yoghurt

- Nuts and nut butters

- Seeds

- Avocados and avocado oil

- Olives and olive oil

- Coconut, coconut milk and coconut oil

- Mayonnaise made with olive oil

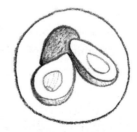

Carbohydrates should provide around 50% of your total calories. When you're looking to add weight, it is definitely not the time to go low-carb, but even if you're bulking, keep added refined sugars as low as possible. There is really nothing to be gained by relying on them. Whole grains, root vegetables, beans, legumes and fruit are where you should get your carbs from – eat lots of them:

- Fresh and dried fruit

- Starchy vegetables like carrots, sweet potatoes, parsnips and squash

- Potatoes and sweet potatoes

- Whole grain bread, bagels, pasta and rice

- Granola

- Trail mix

Weight-gain meal plan

8 a.m.	4 eggs, 2 slices of wholewheat toast, fruit and nut butter smoothie
12.30 p.m.	Chicken curry, rice, broccoli and yoghurt
3 p.m.	Cereal bar or bagel with nut butter
6 p.m.	Steak, sweet potato, green salad with avocado, seeds and olive oil
8 p.m.	Crackers, hummus or nut butter
10 p.m.	Full-fat fruit yoghurt

Weight-gain shakes

At some point, cooking and eating all that food can start to feel like a chore. This is where shakes come in. Weight-gain shakes are similar to other protein shakes, but they are very high in calories – some contain over 1000 calories per serving, whereas protein shakes will normally be around 150 calories per serving and might also include other ingredients that help to build muscles.

You can buy expensive supplement shakes or simply make your own. Making your own with real foods provides more micronutrients and gives your body exactly what it needs. Often, shop-bought shakes are packed with sugar, sweeteners, synthetic nasties and additives with no real nutrients except calories. It literally takes less than a minute to whizz up a delicious shake in your kitchen and bottle it up to take with you.

> ❝ **I was always skinny** and after Tina visited our school I took her advice on how to bulk up. I created a proper meal plan and took my snacks into school, made home-made shakes and really **made the most of every eating window** with better choices. I also started working out at the gym a couple of times a week and I've gained the weight I wanted. I'm never going to be huge, but I do feel much better in myself. ❞
>
> ### HARRY (17)

How to make your own weight-gain shakes

Get creative! Pick at least one ingredient from each category and blend until smooth. Add extra calories any way you can.

Protein	Greek yoghurt, silken tofu, nut butter
Carbs	Any fruits but bananas are best, any grains (like oats, rice or even starchy root veg like cooked sweet potato), honey, molasses or maple syrup
Fats	Nut butters, tahini, avocado, avocado oil
Liquid	Milk, cream, almond milk, coconut milk, coconut water, fruit juice

How to train for weight gain

The formula for gaining weight is really pretty simple: the number of calories you take in must be larger than the number of calories you burn.

Be patient: it may take some time. To get a feeling for how many calories you'll need to put on weight, use an online calculator to determine your total daily energy expenditure (TDEE).

Muscle growth is accelerated with the onset of puberty, between the ages of 13 and 18, and resistance training is key when the goal is to increase muscle mass, size and strength. This can increase muscle weight by up to 15% per year during these years.

If gaining weight is your aim, you need to do three or four strength training sessions a week. This will send your hormones and your muscles a clear message to grow, and it will also increase your appetite. It's not essential to join a gym. You can do bodyweight workouts at home as long as they're demanding enough (there are plenty of videos online to help you get your technique right) and supported by a healthy diet.

A general strengthening programme should address all major muscle groups. For an increase in muscle size, do multiple sets of 8 to 12 repetitions per set. For an increase in power/strength, lift heavier weights and do multiple sets of 4 to 6 reps per set. Heavy weight lifting should always be done under adult supervision.

Rest is an essential part of maintaining a healthy lifestyle.

The body needs to rest in order to rebuild muscle fibres and increase muscle mass. Adolescents should get 8–11 hours of sleep per night.

All about protein

Protein shakes

I get asked all the time about protein shakes and protein bars, and if they are safe. To me, the biggest question is if they are really necessary, even for young athletes. Let me explain. On average, most teenagers need 40–60g of protein per day. Adolescent athletes do need a little more, but most teenagers and young adults get enough protein from food, meaning that supplements are unnecessary and expensive. Recent studies have shown that young athletes consume two to three times the recommended amount of protein per day in their diet.

The best protein sources

The best place to start to increase your protein is to first work on eating more whole food sources like lean meats, fish, tofu, eggs, dairy, beans, legumes, nuts and seeds. You can get the same benefits from introducing high-protein foods to your diet as snacks or adding them to your normal meals to enhance the protein content.

You should aim to eat two to three portions of protein a day and if you're accessing your protein from plant sources, ensure you are eating a wide variety to get all the amino acids and proteins you need (see page 83). I always recommend real food first over shakes. Remember, some of the products on the market are highly processed, often with nasty additives and fillers, and don't contain real nutrients, just calories. It is not uncommon to develop gut issues and acne from protein shakes, especially formulas with whey and casein.

You can work out exactly how much protein you require with a simple calculation. If you're 11–13 years old, multiply your weight in pounds by 0.455; this gives you about how many grams of protein you need each day. For example, a 68kg athlete should consume approximately 70g protein a day ideally, broken into three portions over the duration of the day: 149lb x 0.455 = 70g of protein.

If you're 15–18 years old, multiply your weight in pounds by 0.36 to give you how many grams of protein you need each day. Strength-training athletes may consider using up to 1.4–1.8g of protein per kg a day if needed. Based on a weight of 68kg or 149.6lb, the range would be 95.2–122.4g per day. The table below then helps you work out what foods to eat to achieve the number of grams of protein you need.

What are the effects of protein?

Will eating extra protein make you stronger? No, it won't, because protein supplements don't increase muscle mass, strength or endurance. The amount of protein you consume is irrelevant without the right all-round approach, and the keys to building new muscle are:

- proper training, recovery and sleep

- eating a balance of carbohydrates and protein after exercise

- eating enough calories throughout the day

Too much protein may cause problems, though. Our bodies can't store protein for later use, so it can create stress on the body as it processes it and may well end up down the toilet as you excrete it or it may be converted to fat. Too much protein can cause nausea, loss of appetite, diarrhoea, increase your risk of osteoporosis (a painful bone disease), and can even stress the liver and kidneys. Young bodies are not designed for high-protein, low-carb or low-fat diets.

Ideally, we should aim to eat our protein in small amounts throughout the day, not in one meal, so for example eggs for breakfast, yoghurt for a snack, tuna with lunch and chickpeas for dinner. The magic amount of protein your muscles are capable of absorbing during a meal is 25–35g maximum in any one sitting, so aim for 20–25g of protein as part of the pre- and post-recovery snacks. For example, a 115g serving of chicken, fish or beef provides 25–30g of protein, an egg provides 6g and a glass of milk provides 8g of protein.

Food type	Protein content – g per 100g
Non-plant-based protein	
Half-fat cheddar	32.7
Cheddar	25.4
Chicken breast (grilled without skin)	32.0
Pork chop (lean grilled)	31.6
Beef steak (lean grilled)	31.0
Lamb chop (lean grilled)	29.2
Salmon (grilled)	24.2
Tuna (tinned in brine)	23.5
Prawns	22.6
Cod (grilled)	20.8
Mackerel (grilled)	20.8
Mussels	16.7
Cottage cheese	12.6
Eggs	12.5
Whole milk yoghurt	5.7
Low-fat plain yoghurt	4.8

Semi-skimmed milk	3.4
Skimmed milk	3.4
Whole milk	3.3
Plant-based protein	
Almonds	21.1
Walnuts	14.7
Hazelnuts	14.1
Whole grain flour	12.6
Porridge	11.2
Chickpeas	8.4
Tofu	8.1
Brown bread	7.9
White bread	7.9
Red lentils	7.6
Kidney beans	6.9
Pasta (fresh, cooked)	6.6
Baked beans	5.2
Rice (easy cook, boiled)	2.6

Who might benefit from protein supplements?

If you are an athlete who is vegetarian or vegan, have certain medical conditions or are underweight, you might benefit from protein supplements, after working out whether or not you are getting enough protein from your diet. There are situations where protein supplementation can be very helpful, such as:

- You are recovering from an illness

- You have a poor, weak or unreliable appetite

- You have diet restrictions, allergies, are a fussy eater or have strong food aversion

- You have a very busy schedule that makes it difficult to prep and carry whole food options throughout the day

Whey isolate is generally the most popular protein powder. It is particularly good for recovery as it is the fastest protein to be broken down and absorbed by the body. It also has a lower lactose content, even though it comes from dairy sources, which could be beneficial for those who are lactose intolerant. It undergoes more processing, allowing the protein content to be higher and fat and carbohydrate to be lower, compared to whey concentrate. I also need to mention that whey powders may cause acne as well as stomach issues.

Casein, another protein derived from dairy, is a good 'bedtime' protein option as it is digested slowly throughout the night and continues to aid muscle-building. This is especially helpful if you are unable to consume enough protein throughout the day. Casein can be found in whole food sources too, like cottage cheese and yoghurt. Again, it can increase acne in those with the genetic susceptibility.

Soya and pea protein with a minimal ingredient list are great vegan options. Vegan protein powders that are a mixture of many sources (like pea, soya and rice) are also a great way to help get a blend of essential amino acids.

✳ Summary ✳

If your aim is to gain weight, make every eating opportunity count by ensuring your plate contains proteins, fats and carbohydrates – 50% carbohydrates is the best plate layout for you. A doughnut and junk food diet will not help you gain muscle and the weight you want. Exercise will make you hungrier so incorporate some training into your lifestyle.

To ensure you're eating the right amount of protein, aim for two to three portions of protein a day from fish, shellfish, eggs, dairy, beans or nuts and seeds. If you choose to supplement with a protein powder, look for ones that contain the least number of chemical additives and ideally an organic product. If you find you develop spots or stomach issues, the protein powder may have triggered them, so try a non-dairy option, which will be much easier to tolerate.

Chapter 12

Teenage hormone imbalance

Extreme changes in mood, weight gain and fatigue, and, specifically for girls, facial hair and irregular or heavy periods are all common symptoms of teenage hormone imbalance, but there are other less common signs as well and these can occur in various combinations, depending on your specific hormonal issues.

Less common signs for girls

- Periods that last longer than a week
- Heavy menstrual bleeding requiring a pad or tampon change every two to three hours
- Severe cramping
- Hair growth on the chin or lower belly
- Hair loss on the head
- Unexplained weight gain

- Extreme fatigue

- Dry skin

- Puffy or rounded face

- Extreme mood swings, depression or anxiety

- Increased sensitivity to heat or cold

Less common signs for boys

- Gynaecomastia or the development of breast tissue

- Breast tenderness

- Erectile dysfunction

- Decrease in beard and body hair growth

- Loss of muscle mass

- Loss of bone mass (osteoporosis)

- Difficulty concentrating

- Hot flushes

Hormones that cause girls problems

Oestrogen is a hormone that has various roles to play in the body. In girls and women, it helps develop and maintain the reproductive system, breasts and pubic hair. It also contributes to brain, bone and heart health, and other essential bodily processes.

Progesterone, which is made by the ovaries, is another hormone whose main function is regulating menstruation and supporting pregnancy. Irregular periods, headaches and anxiety can be caused by low levels of progesterone, but it also has an important role in balancing oestrogen.

If progesterone is low, oestrogen can by contrast be too high, creating other issues, such as PMS, mood swings, tender breasts, loss of sex drive and weight gain. Low oestrogen, on the other hand, can cause tiredness, lack of concentration, urine infections and hot flushes.

As a teenage girl, another hormone you need to know about is cortisol, often nicknamed the 'stress hormone'. If your cortisol levels are too high it can cause anxiety, depression and weight gain, while weight loss and tiredness can be a product of low cortisol levels.

Foods to help balance female hormones

Adding healthy fats like monounsaturated fats such as olive oil and avocado or omega-3 to your diet will help support your hormone balance, which can help high or low oestrogen levels. High-quality omega-3 fats include:

- Mackerel, wild salmon, wild trout, herring, anchovies
- Walnuts
- Chia seeds
- Flaxseeds
- Algae oil supplements

Other foods to boost oestrogen levels include:

- Alfalfa sprouts
- Dried fruit
- Eggs
- Fennel
- Garlic
- Hummus
- Sesame seeds
- Soya beans/edamame beans
- Tofu
- Wholegrain bread

Certain foods can help to support progesterone production by balancing oestrogen (walnuts, cabbage, shellfish) and stimulating progesterone production (beans, sesame, broccoli, pumpkin, kale, spinach). Also ensure you are consuming vitamin B- and vitamin C-rich foods every day – the body doesn't store either of these and they are essential for the balanced levels of progesterone and oestrogen. You can find vitamin B in:

- Milk
- Cheese
- Eggs
- Meat, such as chicken and red meat
- Fish, such as tuna, mackerel and salmon
- Shellfish, such as prawns, mussels and scallops
- Dark green vegetables, such as spinach and kale

The following are good sources of vitamin C:

- Kiwis
- Citrus fruit
- Peppers
- Berries
- Leafy green vegetables

Hormones that cause boys problems

For teenage boys, zinc and vitamin D deficiency is very common (white spots on your nails are a sure sign that you are deficient in zinc), but without these you won't be able to produce testosterone effectively. Testosterone is a sex hormone and in men it's thought to regulate sex drive (libido) and is needed for sperm and red blood cell production, as well as for muscle mass and strength.

Foods to help balance male hormones

If your overall diet is healthy, you should get plenty of the nutrients your body needs to grow and function properly, but foods where you can find zinc and vitamin D include:

- Fish, such as tuna, salmon and white fish

- Shellfish, such as prawns, mussels, scallops and crab

- Eggs

- Milk

- Yoghurt

- Cheese

- Beans, such as baked beans, chickpeas and lentils

In very rare cases (just 2%) teen boys may have delayed puberty. If you are an older teen (14+) and not yet showing any signs of starting puberty, you can go to your GP and discuss having an injection of small amounts of testosterone to kick-start puberty. However, whenever possible it is best to let the body begin producing the hormones you need on its own.

And a word about cortisol, which is commonly called the 'stress hormone' and has a vital role in your body's response to stress (for more on dealing with stress, see page 158). After your body releases its 'fight or flight' hormones, such as adrenaline, it then releases cortisol, so you stay on high alert. Very high levels of cortisol may make boys (and girls too) crave fatty, sugary and starchy foods, resulting in weight gain. Low levels of cortisol are very rare, but symptoms include fatigue, dizziness (especially when you stand up), weight loss, muscle weakness, mood changes and dark patches on your skin.

Common causes of female hormone imbalance

If you experience irregular or heavy periods, it's possible you may have a condition called polycystic ovary syndrome (PCOS). Other symptoms are acne, excessive body hair, patches of dark skin and weight gain.

Doctors aren't exactly sure what causes PCOS, but hormone imbalance is thought to be a factor, although there may also be a genetic component, meaning that if someone in your family has it, you may be at risk too. If you have these symptoms, it's best to go and see your doctor.

We do know, though, that exposure to environmental toxins has an impact on causing imbalances in our hormones. For example, many environmental chemicals, known as xenoestrogens, can affect a developing hormone system.

Xenoestrogens

Did you know that what you put on your skin, the largest organ in our body, is absorbed and travels through our bloodstream? Many self-care and beauty products, as well as household cleaning products, contain synthetic chemicals that can disrupt our hormone system by mimicking oestrogen in our bodies, leading to 'oestrogen dominance'. Always check the label of any products you use, and aim to go for paraben-free and natural products.

Xenoestrogens in the environment

- Plastics – water bottles, disposable cups, cling film, food containers

- Pesticides – on non-organic fruits and vegetables

- Tap water – chlorine and other chemical treatments (but using a water filter can improve water quality)

- Chemicals in cosmetics, lotions, shampoos and other body care products

- Birth control pills

Xenoestrogens in plastics

- Cut back on your use of plastic wherever you can

- Don't refill plastic water bottles

- Don't freeze water in plastic water bottles

- Don't leave plastic water bottles in the sun

- Don't put packed lunches in plastic bags

- Don't use cling film to cover or microwave food

- Don't microwave food in plastic containers

Xenoestrogens in health and beauty products

- Use toothpastes and soaps that don't contain harmful ingredients

- Choose eco-friendly period products like period pants or plastic-free tampons

- Opt for natural fragrances like essential oils

- Avoid cosmetics and creams containing toxic chemicals and ingredients such as parabens

- Only use nail varnish and nail varnish removers occasionally

Natural ways to regulate oestrogen levels in the body

- Drink more water, because this helps get rid of excess oestrogen in your body

- Do a poo every day if you can as this also helps excrete excess oestrogen

- Eat broccoli, kale, cabbage and Brussels sprouts as they can help reduce the effects of oestrogen and support the liver's detox function. Try a homemade chunky slaw

- Keep your alcohol and caffeine intake low to support your kidney, liver and natural detox processes

- Regular exercise helps you lose excess oestrogen too

- Avoid processed and refined carbohydrates and sugar, which can increase oestrogen and result in weight gain

What treatments are there for hormone imbalance in both boys and girls?

Excess hormones need to be metabolised (broken down) by the liver, excreted through our gut and disposed of when we do a poo. Some basic principles are to ensure you're eating a healthy, fibre-rich, balanced diet every day. Fibre from fruits, vegetables, whole grains, beans, pulses, nuts and seeds help bind to oestrogen and ensure it exits through our bowels.

Fat is essential for hormone production and balance. I recommend a diet high in healthy fats like omega-3s and monounsaturated fats for those who are suffering from hormonal imbalance.

Certain foods can help to support progesterone production by reducing oestrogen (walnuts, cabbage, shellfish) or stimulating progesterone production (beans, sesame, broccoli, pumpkin, kale and spinach).

Hydration and daily movement or exercise are both important to ensure that you get your bowels moving each day, which aids excretion and the elimination of toxins and excess hormones. If this doesn't happen, the hormones recirculate in your body.

Once you've corrected your diet, the next issue that must be addressed is the bacterial balance in the digestive system. Try adding some fermented foods like kefir, sauerkraut or kombucha, which can help improve the health of the gut.

The next piece of the puzzle is correcting the underlying hormone imbalance. To do this, you must first limit your sugar intake, because sugar directly disrupts the hormone balance and reduces the liver's ability to metabolise or process our hormones.

Too much sugar leads to too much insulin and high levels of this particular hormone can affect the normal workings of a women's ovaries, resulting in the production of the hormone testosterone. Higher levels of testosterone can affect the development of follicles, raise the likelihood of PCOS (see page 118), cause PMS and affect the regularity of periods, as well as causing excess body hair and acne.

While excess sugar in the diet can raise testosterone levels in women, it may lower testosterone levels in men, leading to lower libido and erectile dysfunction as well as obesity and diabetes. For both men and women, insulin production can inhibit the production of human growth hormone, which is responsible for optimal muscle mass, body fat and bone structure.

Ever heard of the adrenal glands? These are where we produce our stress hormones like cortisol and adrenalin. Teens suffer a lot from stress and elevated cortisol from stress disrupts the balance in the endocrine system, the system of glands that produces hormones. Again, exercise is a great stress-releaser so try to get some exercise every day or try things like yoga and breathing exercises to de-stress.

The power of sleep! Constant stimulation is not healthy for our adrenal glands and sufficient sleep is essential.

Our body does a lot of its detoxing when we're sleeping, and sleep also rejuvenates organs like our liver, so they are more effective at their job, so prioritise getting sufficient sleep and make sure you allow time each day for a digital detox.

Keep calm and cope with your PMS

Premenstrual syndrome (PMS) is the physical, psychological and behavioural symptoms that often occur in the days before a monthly period. Also known as premenstrual tension (PMT), symptoms vary from person to person, but typically occur in the two weeks before the period starts, improving and easing once the period starts and in the days after.

There have been more than 100 different symptoms of PMS recorded. Generally, symptoms of PMS fall into two categories: physical, and psychological and behavioural. Common physical symptoms include:

- bloating

- headaches

- backache

- breast pain

- tummy pain and discomfort

- sleeping problems

- weight gain (up to 1kg)

Common psychological and behavioural symptoms include:

- mood swings

- emotional

- irritable

- difficulty concentrating

- clumsiness

- tiredness

- restlessness

- decreased self-esteem

- food cravings and/or appetite changes

Any long-term conditions, such as asthma or migraines, may get worse during this time. Certain lifestyle factors are thought to worsen symptoms, such as lack of exercise, poor diet and stress, and, while lifestyle changes won't make PMS disappear, they can help to ease symptoms, making the days and weeks before your cycle begins more manageable.

Of course, regular physical activity is essential in maintaining a healthy lifestyle. If possible, aim to do at least 150 minutes of moderate-intensity activity each week (30 minutes for five days). This could be walking, swimming or cycling. Regular exercise keeps the body healthy and can also help alleviate tiredness and depression. Stretching-based activities, such as yoga and Pilates, are great ways to de-stress and help you sleep better. In some cases, stretching is also thought to help ease abdominal discomfort during your period.

How nutrition can help alleviate PMT

Changes in hormone levels are thought to be a primary cause of PMT. Therefore, a fibre-rich diet can be highly beneficial for those with severe symptoms. This is because fibre reduces the stress on your liver – the organ that metabolises hormones, including oestrogen. Furthermore, once digested, fibre absorbs excess oestrogen and transports it out of the body. The added benefit is that fibre balances blood sugar, which can help to control mood swings and fatigue. Now let's look at some foods that can help prevent PMT.

Essential fatty acids

Eating foods rich in essential fatty acids (such as mixed nuts, seeds, oily fish, avocados, olive oil and seed oils) can make a big difference to PMT symptoms. This is because essential fatty acids help regulate hormones and reduce inflammation.

Foods rich in vitamin B6

Bananas, whole grains, eggs, beans and nuts are among the foods that contain vitamin B6. This vitamin is effective not only for pain relief, but it can also help the liver to remove excess oestrogen. Research also shows a link between vitamin B6 and reduced depression and irritability.

Natural live yoghurt

Research suggests women who eat a diet rich in calcium have a 40% lower risk of developing PMT. Just a small pot of natural yoghurt contains 25% of your daily recommended intake of calcium, which makes it a great snack option for tackling PMT symptoms.

Camomile tea

Camomile tea in your diet could make a huge difference to your PMT symptoms. This is because it contains antispasmodic properties that can help to ease the severity of menstrual cramps and muscle spasms. Camomile tea is also highly relaxing and can help to soothe stress and anxiety.

Other nutrients to help with your hormonal balance

Magnesium is naturally calming and helps us feel relaxed – you could call it nature's tranquilliser! Enjoy an Epsom salts bath a couple of times a week. Put two mugs of Epsom salts into your bathwater and enjoy a warm soak for at least 20 minutes. We absorb magnesium very well through our skin. The reason so many of us crave chocolate so much the week before our period is because it is another great source of magnesium. While there's no reason not to enjoy some antioxidant-rich dark chocolate, try to up your intake of this essential mineral from foods such as green leafy veg (spinach, watercress, kale), nuts and seeds (flax, pumpkin), legumes (beans, chickpeas and lentils) and whole grains.

Diets low in vitamins B1, B2 and B6 are associated with a higher occurrence of PMS. B1 can be found in fortified cereals, legumes and nuts, and B2 can be found in cow's milk, red meat and leafy green vegetables, while tuna, salmon, chicken and chickpeas are all good sources of B6. B12 is yet another one that plays a major role in emotional stability, but it is only available from animal products, so if you are a vegan you should take a B12 supplement.

Vitamin D is a very common nutrient to be deficient in during the winter months, but girls with high levels of vitamin D are less likely to have PMS symptoms. Try vitamin D drops or a mouth spray throughout the winter months, from October to April.

Again, women whose diet is rich in calcium are less likely to suffer PMS. Three servings of dairy products (one yoghurt, some cheese, a glass of milk) are recommended each day to supply enough of this nutrient. If you don't enjoy dairy products, calcium can also be found in almonds, dried fruits such as figs and apricots, and leafy green vegetables like broccoli, cabbage and kale. Make sure you are eating some of these every day.

Phytoestrogens from foods such as tofu, edamame beans, lentils, oats, barley, flaxseeds, sesame seeds, almonds and pistachios can help balance your hormones and may reduce PMS symptoms such as headaches.

✳ Summary ✳

For all teenagers, nutrient deficiencies and hormone disrupters such as xenoestrogens can create hormone imbalances. Specific foods and nutrients can help balance our hormones, and exercise and other lifestyle factors also play a part in ensuring we maintain a happy hormone balance.

For girls, symptoms of PMS can be really troublesome, but there are lots of things that can help improve your symptoms in the lead-up to your period. A combination of targeted nutrition, by including certain foods, along with exercise and relaxation techniques has the power to dramatically improve how you feel.

Chapter 13

How to get more ZZZs

Just think of all the things you cram into your day: school, sports, hobbies, walking pets, running around and seeing friends, and homework. By the end of every day, is it any wonder your body needs to rest?

Without a good night's sleep, we can feel groggy, lethargic and just not our best. When we don't sleep well we can experience mood changes, feel overwhelmed and have difficulty concentrating (aka brain fog). Our immune function can be compromised too.

We're also likely to eat more and we're likely to crave more sugary foods. Sleep deprivation increases the hunger hormone ghrelin and decreases the satiety (feeling of fullness) hormone leptin. This means that when you haven't slept well you need more food to have the same effect on your appetite, so lack of sleep makes us eat more food and crave more carbohydrate foods, and therefore affects our weight and waistline.

WHY DO WE NEED SO MUCH SLEEP?

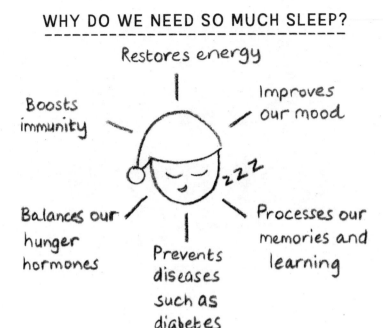

Restores energy

Boosts immunity

Improves our mood

Balances our hunger hormones

Prevents diseases such as diabetes

Processes our memories and learning

So how much is enough sleep? If you're 13 to 17 years old you need eight to ten hours a night, whereas 18 to 25-year-olds need a little less – seven to nine hours – and pre-teens need a little more with nine to 11 hours a night.

Circadian rhythms and sleep

Circadian rhythms are physical, mental, and behavioural changes that follow a 24-hour cycle. These natural processes respond primarily to light and dark, and affect most living things, including humans, animals and plants. They effectively form our sleep/wake cycle or what is also referred to as our biological clock, which is our natural timing device, regulating the cycle of circadian rhythms.

In order for it to make melatonin to sleep well and stay asleep, and to switch off melatonin production in the morning, so that you don't feel groggy and sleepy during the day, studies show that your body needs sunlight (blue light) as soon as you rise and total darkness at night. If you sleep with the light on, your sleep will be shallow and you will wake up frequently, but the light will also affect your brain waves, particularly those related to deep sleep.

It really is important to try to get outside and see natural daylight as soon as you wake up. Don't leave your curtains closed when you wake up in the morning as this will prevent your body from creating the natural sleep/wake cycle.

AVERAGE TEENAGE CIRCADIAN CYCLE

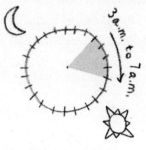

Dropping off
Once you're asleep, your energy levels drop right down and are at their lowest between about 3a.m. and 7a.m.. You may not feel properly awake again until 9a.m. or even 10a.m..

On high alert
During the morning your body temperature rises steadily and so do your energy levels. In fact, you should feel noticeably sharp and on the ball right up to lunchtime.

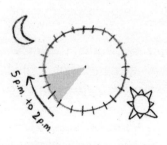

Afternoon slump
Everyone tends to get hit by this, but as a teenager you woke up later so you'll experience an energy dip later than most adults, some time between 2p.m. and 5p.m..

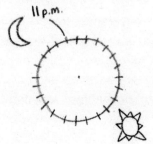

Feeling tired
It's not surprising you want to stay up later than your parents and past 11p.m., because the sleep hormone, melatonin, kicks in about an hour later for teenagers than it does for adults.

> **I couldn't sleep.** *I found it almost impossible to switch off at night and I would wake up regularly and find it hard to get back to sleep. Then I started waking up early every morning, was always grumpy and couldn't cope with school. When I went to see Tina I learnt all about how important it is to get* **sunlight first thing in the morning** *and how caffeine and the way I was eating was causing a lot of blood sugar and sleeping problems. I always felt a bit stressed and wired and Tina taught me techniques to wind down and switch off.*

TOBY (17)

LIGHT UP MY LIFE

Exposure to natural light first thing plays an important role in regulating the sleep-inducing hormone, melatonin, which the body releases at night to help you get to sleep. Morning light suppresses melatonin, so your body wakes up, and it also boosts serotonin, a brain chemical that can make you feel more energetic, positive and focused.

Due to the lack of light, particularly sunshine, during the winter months, some people suffer from a type of depression called seasonal affective disorder (SAD). However, this can be treated with natural and artificial light.

Daylight has a very direct effect on the body, boosting bone-strengthening vitamin D and lifting your mood. A walk outdoors will get your circulation going, improve your concentration and clear your head. Perhaps start walking to school or get off the bus a stop or two earlier, so you can walk a bit more.

Fresh air and exercise are just as important as sleep and good nutrition. We are like plants. Without fresh air, sunlight and good nutrition, we will feel ourselves wilt and no longer thrive, so what are you waiting for? Get outside!

Make sure all your screen displays are set to night-time settings to prevent them emitting strong blue light in the evening. If you struggle with getting to sleep, it may be that you are letting in too much blue light in the evening. You can buy blue-light-blocking glasses or simply try winding down without screens in the evening an hour or two before you want to sleep. Enjoy a bath, try meditating or doing yoga, or swap your book for an eReader like a Kindle Paperwhite, which allows you to read without using a light.

THE MICROBIOME AND SLEEP

Growing evidence suggests that the gut microbiome can influence sleep quality. Studies show that good bacterial/microbial diversity is associated with improved sleep quality and duration, and promotes healthier sleep (for more about how to feed your gut bacteria, see page 32).

What can you eat to help you sleep?

Melatonin, the sleep hormone, is produced from the foods we eat, so for us to sleep well we need to consume certain nutrients. Fibre from vegetables, wholegrains, beans and legumes provides the best fuel for our gut bacteria, which actually makes the melatonin, but it needs vitamin B6, which is in bananas, and fish like tuna and salmon, and the amino acid tryptophan, found in chicken, turkey, carbohydrates, dairy, nuts and seeds.

Magnesium, found in leafy green vegetables, whole grains, and nuts and seeds, helps with muscle and nerve relaxation, and calcium, for example from leafy vegetables like kale, is also required. Milk itself contains melatonin, which is why it is sometimes recommended to help you get to sleep.

If you're vegetarian or vegan you need to make sure that you're eating foods rich in all these important nutrients, and low levels of omega-3, present in oily fish, are also associated with poorer sleep quality, so you may want to think about taking an algae omega-3 supplement (see page 80).

Studies showed that people who ate oily fish a couple of times a week had better overall sleep as well as improved daytime functioning. Other research found that eating kiwi can improve sleep. In a study, people who ate two kiwis an hour before bed found that they fell asleep faster, slept more and had better-quality sleep.

For a good sleep, aim for an evening meal containing a combination of a moderate amount of tryptophan-rich protein and some slow-release complex carbohydrates, which will make it easier for the tryptophan to reach the brain. A banana and some warm milk or a yoghurt with nuts and seeds both make good pre-bedtime snacks.

How to sleep better

If you struggle with sleep, here are some top tips to help you improve it:

- Try to go to bed at the same time every night as this helps the body get into a routine
- Follow a calming bedtime routine, such as taking a warm shower or reading
- Deep breathing exercises will have a calming effect on your body – breathe in for four seconds, hold for four seconds and breathe out for eight seconds
- Try putting lavender oil on your pillow
- Limit foods that contain caffeine and sugar, including chocolate, fizzy drinks, energy drinks, hot chocolate and tea
- Try drinking a small cup of sleepy-time tea, which includes calming herbs such as camomile, valerian or passionflower, half an hour before you want to go to sleep
- If you're hungry you may not be able to sleep, so try a bedtime snack

- Skipping carbohydrates or reducing your calorie intake can make you sleep badly – to induce sleep, trying upping the carbohydrates in your evening meal to at least a third to a half of your plate

- Magnesium is a natural tranquilliser and great to help you sleep. It's absorbed well through the skin – you can buy magnesium oil from the chemist to rub on your inner arms or thighs or have a soak in an Epsom salts bath for 20–30 minutes (put two small mugs of Epsom salts into hot running water)

- Make sure your room is very dark – try an eye mask if you don't have blackout curtains or there is too much light coming in

- If you find it too noisy, try wax earplugs to cut out the noise

- Don't watch scary TV shows or movies close to bedtime, because these can make it hard to fall asleep

- Don't exercise just before bed unless it is gentle yoga

- Use your bed just for sleeping – not doing homework, reading, playing games or talking on the phone – so you'll train your body to associate your bed only with sleeping

- If you are really struggling, try using calming sleep or meditation apps

- Try blue-light-blocking glasses if you have long-term problems getting to sleep

SETTING YOURSELF UP FOR THE DAY

- Set your alarm with 5–10 minutes to spare in bed
- Avoid the snooze button
- Avoid looking at your phone or social media instantly
- Rehydrate
- Get moving/stretch
- Opt for a protein-rich balanced breakfast
- Allow natural light in the room

∗ Summary ∗

Sleep is crucial and has a specific role in memory consolidation during learning and revision. Poor sleep and sleep deficit are linked to poor attention and cognition. Lack of sleep also affects our mood, weight, blood sugar regulation appetite and skin health. **Prioritise sleep to ensure that you stay well,** to optimise your cognitive performance and to maintain a healthy weight. People with insomnia and depression may have low levels of healthy gut bacteria. More research on this topic is required.

Chapter 14

Build a healthy relationship with food

Creating healthy habits and eating well doesn't mean not enjoying treat foods and social events with friends. Try to eat well Monday to Friday – 70 to 80% of the time – by ensuring you're eating three balanced meals and snacks if you need them each day. Then at the weekends – 20 to 30% of the time – you can be more relaxed, go out for pizza with your friends or enjoy chocolate brownies for treats. For the 20%, you needn't worry about whether meals or snacks are balanced. You've eaten so well during the week that your nutritional status will still be excellent. This is the 80:20 rule we looked at earlier in the book.

No such thing as bad or good foods

There really is no such thing as good or bad, or superfoods. It's important not to demonise foods or be scared of food. However, all foods are not necessarily equal in terms of how they make you feel. Learning to listen to your body and how it responds to different foods is really helpful. For instance, do you find you get a big energy dip after eating really sugary food? If that happens to you, here's a tip: try eating it after a meal as the protein and fibre from the meal will reduce the sugar spike.

Becoming obsessed with 'healthy' eating can be a problem as it can be limiting and, in many ways, isolating. You may start to worry about what you will be eating when, and if all the food is 'healthy' at school or whenever you're eating out.

Having balance around eating well is about understanding that we can't control our environment or the food we eat 100% of the time, nor should we try to. Know that if we aim to eat well 70 to 80% of the time, there is no need to worry about other times when we can't choose what we eat.

> **Eating for well-being focuses on individualised eating based on hunger, satiety, nutritional needs and pleasure, rather than concentrating on weight control.**

Socialising and food

Socialising and food have been closely linked through history, and this tradition is passed down through the ages from one generation to the next. We want to be able to participate in social events and occasions without fear of what food will be served.

Equally, in our Western society, where we have an abundance of highly calorific food available to us, and we socialise, get takeaways and eat in restaurants more than ever, we may find that we can put on extra weight we don't want.

Instead, try creating your own healthier takeaway meals – for example, home-cooked Nando's, healthy biscuits or the black bean brownies on page 216 – rather than ordering high-calorie Domino's pizza and consuming fizzy drinks.

It's also important to recognise that when we socialise it doesn't always have to include eating and to acknowledge that the most important reason to socialise has nothing to do with food. You don't need food to interact with people you like to spend time with. Try creating more active social activities. Meet up and go for a walk, run or cycle. Perhaps enjoy swimming together. Or simply invite friends over to chat rather than to eat.

❝ I had a really difficult relationship with food. *I'd either binge-eat – literally eating anything I could get my hands on – or starve myself. This way of eating led me to have low moods and I no longer felt motivated to do my college work a lot of the time. However, when I learnt about how food affects every aspect of our bodies, slowly, over several months, I started to eat better and feel better, and I was able to enjoy college a lot more.* **I also enjoy being able to sleep** *– I think I was often too hungry and couldn't sleep – and more sleep means I just have much more energy.* ❞

SHILPA (17)

How to control overeating

Many of us eat way too much food and find it difficult to control our appetites, especially with today's ever-increasing portion sizes, and access to high-calorie foods and snacks just about everywhere we go. What's more, when we eat high-sugar or white processed foods (bread, pasta, rice, biscuits, cakes, chocolate bars, sweets and sugary drinks), this drives our hunger hormones and can create an insatiable appetite.

One of the easiest ways to make sure that we eat well, but don't overeat, is to create a simple meal plan, so that we ensure we include all the important food groups each day and over the entire week. Use this as an outline to create your own menu plan or get the whole family involved. On the following pages, there is an example covering seven days' worth of meals:

	Day 1	Day 2	Day 3	Day 4	Day 5	Day 6	Day 7
Breakfast	2 scrambled eggs, 1 or 2 slices wholegrain toast, piece of fruit, palm-sized portion of unsalted mixed nuts or seeds	Bowl of porridge with half a chopped or grated apple and cinnamon or stewed apple and cinnamon, with 2 tsp ground flax or mixed seeds, piece of fruit, palm-sized portion of unsalted mixed nuts or seeds	Homemade Bircher muesli with yoghurt, oats with grated apple or berries and seeds, piece of fruit, palm-sized portion of unsalted mixed nuts or seeds	Greek yoghurt, granola, piece of fruit, palm-sized portion of unsalted mixed nuts or seeds	Hummus, wholegrain pitta, home-made smoothie with frozen berries, plain yoghurt and a little water, piece of fruit, palm-sized portion of unsalted mixed nuts or seeds	Grilled chicken sausages, low-sugar baked beans, wholegrain toast, piece of fruit, palm-sized portion of unsalted mixed nuts or seeds	Avocado and tomato on sourdough or rye bread, piece of fruit, palm-sized portion of unsalted mixed nuts or seeds
Snack	Oatcakes with hummus piece of fruit	Hummus and carrot sticks, piece of fruit	Oatcakes or brown rice cakes, smoked mackerel pâté, piece of fruit	Rye crackers, oatcakes or brown rice cakes, cheese spread or nut butter or hummus, piece of fruit	Plum, apricot or satsuma, low-sugar ginger biscuits	Carrot cake	Seeded flapjack, piece of fruit

Lunch	Bowl of chunky lentil and vegetable soup, wholemeal or granary roll and butter, cheese	Pasta, tinned wild salmon and fresh tomato sauce, broccoli or mixed salad	Savoury couscous, roasted courgettes, peppers, onions and herbs, chickpeas or chicken, salad	Baked potato, tuna and sweetcorn or low-sugar baked beans, salad greens	Thai chicken, prawn or veggie curry (including green veg), egg-fried wild and basmati rice, broccoli, wilted green leafy veg	Two- or three-egg vegetable frittata, green leafy veg or salad	Roast chicken, roasted vegetables including sweet potato, gravy, fruit crumble and crème fraiche
Snack	Chopped crudités, wholemeal pitta, hummus or baba ghanoush	Seeded flapjack, piece of fruit	Natural yoghurt with added fruit or energy balls	Apple or pear with nut butter	Rye crackers with smoked mackerel	Energy balls	Banana bread
Dinner	Salmon fishcakes, sweet potatoes, broccoli	Stir-fry tofu, chicken noodles or brown rice, shredded veg, beansprouts, ginger and spring onions, soya sauce	Baked haddock in cheese sauce, sweet potato mash, steamed veg	Egg-fried brown and white basmati rice, prawns, peas, sweetcorn, peppers and broccoli	Seared chicken or mixed bean and pepper fajitas, carrot and raisin salad with olive oil and balsamic	Vegetable, five-bean or lentil chilli con carne, quinoa, green beans	Soft-boiled eggs, wholemeal soldiers, asparagus spears, chopped fruit

Here is a simple vegetarian or pescatarian eight-day meal plan (for snacks, use the omnivore meal plan for inspiration):

	Day 1	Day 2	Day 3	Day 4	Day 5	Day 6	Day 7	Day 8
Break-fast	Porridge, fruit and nuts	Greek yoghurt, muesli, blue-berries	Nut butter on wholegrain sourdough bread, piece of fruit	Mushroom omelette, piece of fruit	Avocado and tomatoes on sourdough, satsuma	Smoked salmon and cucumber on wholegrain bagel, piece of fruit	Overnight oats, pears and nuts	Hummus and wholegrain pitta, fruit
Lunch	Red lentil and bean burger, sweet potato fries, salad	Pasta, tinned wild salmon and fresh tomato sauce, broc-coli	Cheese, asparagus and pea baked pasta	Rolled auber-gine stuffed with ricotta and spinach, tomato and basil sauce, salad	Bean and brown rice quesadillas, chunky slaw, sour cream, salsa	Falafel salad, pitta, tahini dressing. berries and yoghurt	Quorn burger, leftover rice and vegeta-bles	Veggie and lentil soup, bread, cheese, pieces of fruit
Dinner	Mozzarella or vegan feta, basil and courgette frittata	Butternut squash and black bean tortilla wraps, guacamole	Gnocchi, pesto, broc-coli, tinned wild salmon or chick-peas	Vegetarian tikka masala, black-eyed beans	Goan fish, butternut squash and butter bean curry, brown rice, vegeta-bles	Egg-fried rice with prawns or tofu and vegetables	Mac and cheese, Swiss chard	Tex-mex black bean and quinoa bowl, shredded slaw

Count your nutrients, not your calories. Ditch restricted diets and think about what you can add into your diet to help you THRIVE! Focus on <u>nourishing yourself</u> physically, mentally and emotionally, and consider how food makes you FEEL!

Creating a meal plan also ensures that we know what we will eat the majority of the time, and that we have snacks with us to sustain us should we get hungry, rather than grabbing a pack of crisps and a chocolate bar on the run.

The biggest key to keeping healthy and eating well is to understand about healthy eating and to be able to create simple healthy meals in minutes. Try to cook new recipes (see page 175) as often as possible, so that you become confident in the kitchen, and use some of the following strategies too.

Eat slowly

It takes about 20 minutes for the brain to realise that the stomach is full and to give the cue that you should stop eating. Taking more time to eat, and chewing each mouthful properly, gives your brain plenty of time to send that signal and, if you feel full, you'll eat less.

TOP TIP

→ Some people need to eat just three times a day and they don't get hungry or tired between meals. However, if you find you get energy lows mid-morning and afternoon, you may be better off eating three smaller meals and two snacks. ←

Watch healthy portion sizes

The difference between the average waistline size now and in the 1950s has gone from 61cm to an average 87cm waist. Why the dramatic increase in our waistlines? This is due to several factors, such as access to highly processed, addictive foods, less exercise in our daily lives and a huge difference in our portion sizes. Just eating slightly smaller portions (see page 30) can ensure you stay a healthy weight effortlessly!

Remove temptation

It is hard to stick to a meal plan when the cupboard is full of all your favourite treat foods. Don't keep your cupboards stocked with treats such as crisps, chocolate and sweets. Create a time each week when you will enjoy treats. For example, perhaps on Saturdays you buy and enjoy some sweets, rather than having access to them every day.

Avoid last-minute food choices

Making last-minute meal and snack decisions is a common trigger for overeating. When we make impulsive food choices, it can be easy to pick nutritionally poor, calorie-dense foods or order takeaways.

Eat high-fibre foods

We know that the more fibre we eat, the fuller we feel for longer. Fibre is a type of plant carbohydrate that occurs in many foods, including whole grains, beans, peas and lentils, many vegetables, nuts and seeds, and fruit, including the skins. Here are some ideas for ways to eat more fibre:

- Avocado on wholegrain toast or rye crackers
- Chia and fruit pots
- Porridge with added seeds
- Lentil and vegetable soup
- Dhal and brown rice
- Tuna sandwich with wholegrain bread
- Jacket potatoes and baked beans
- Bean chilli and brown rice
- Roasted chickpeas
- Oatcakes and hummus
- Rye crackers with cheese
- Home-made trail mix
- Peanut butter on a chopped apple

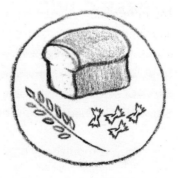

Eat protein-rich foods

Protein-rich foods tend to create a longer-lasting sense of fullness and satisfaction than other foods. Eating protein-rich foods, especially at breakfast, reduces the effect of our hunger hormone, ghrelin. High-protein foods and snacks include high-protein yoghurts and yoghurt drinks, nuts and seeds, full fat milk and cheese, beans, lentils and peas, for example hummus, fish, poultry, beef, eggs and tofu.

Stay hydrated

Ensuring that you're hydrated is a very helpful way to prevent overeating. Our trigger for thirst can be confused with hunger, so if you are always hungry, look to your water intake first.

Find your trigger

Work out the cause of your overeating. Many of us have trigger foods that make us overeat. I love baguettes with butter. I know that I could easily eat a whole large baguette, so rather than buying baguettes, I choose to buy smaller individual wholegrain rolls, which don't trigger me to overeat. Make a list of foods that you find trigger overeating and eat them just occasionally.

When our relationship with food breaks down...

It can be very stressful to worry about food and heathy eating all the time, which is what someone with orthorexia nervosa does. Like anorexia nervosa or bulimia nervosa, it can be described as an eating disorder. Signs that someone might be orthorexic are:

- They compulsively check nutrition labels and ingredient lists
- They cut out an increasing number of food groups (all sugar, all carbs, all dairy, all meat, all animal products)

- They become distressed when 'healthy' foods aren't available

- They take an unusual interest in how healthy the food other people are eating is

- They spend a lot of time thinking about the food being served at future events

- They may or may not have body image concerns

There's a fine line between eating more healthily, which is obviously a good thing, and becoming obsessed with consuming only 'healthy', 'pure' or 'clean' food. If someone becomes obsessed like this, it can result in malnutrition and, sometimes, heart issues and other problems related to malnutrition. They may perceive themselves as 'pure' and other people as 'impure', which can test friendships and may leave them socially isolated. If you feel that you may be orthorexic, please talk to a medical professional, because there is help available and you don't have to live like this.

All about eating disorders

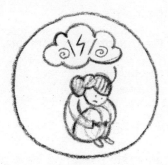

Food is a vital part of our daily lives and many of us spend a significant part of our day thinking about our next meal. However, if signs of obsessive behaviour towards eating or controlling the food you eat arise, then it may be a problem.

It is often believed that to have an eating disorder you must be either overweight or underweight. This is not the case. Anybody, no matter what their size, age or gender, can be diagnosed with an eating disorder.

Teenagers who go on fad or crash diets put themselves at serious risk by not eating enough for their development. It is incredibly important for healthy mental and physical development that you feed yourselves enough to fuel changes and growth. Serious dieting and restrictive eating can lead to poor concentration, fatigue and loss of muscle and bone density, and it's also common to experience changes in mood and personality.

Dieting can also develop into serious eating disorders such as anorexia nervosa or bulimia nervosa, both of which are also serious mental health disorders. Some signs to be aware of include: binge-eating, avoiding food, repetitive dieting, repetitive weighing and excessive exercising.

If you have an eating problem, you might:

- Obsess about food constantly

- Eat as an emotional response even if you don't feel hungry

- Have very specific rules about eating (and become very upset when they're broken)

- Feel anxious about eating

- Be unable to bear the thought of certain foods

- Control how much food you eat

- Much prefer to eat in secret

- Get rid of what you eat (purging)

- Weigh yourself frequently (equating how much you weigh with self-worth)

What it's like to have an eating issue

Eating issues are not just about food. You may have painful feelings that you find hard to express, face or resolve. Controlling what and how you eat may be a way of disguising these problems, even from yourself.

You may notice your friends and loved ones mentioning the changes that eating problems have had on your body. However, it is possible that they don't notice at all, because your body looks different to how they believe someone with an eating disorder should look.

It is also possible to have eating problems and keep them hidden, sometimes for a very long time. And it is also very common to not know yourself if your complicated relationship with eating is a 'real' problem. This is often because the struggles have become ingrained into your everyday life. Some people refuse to seek help, because they don't think their problem is serious enough or that they are not 'good enough' at their eating problem.

There is plenty of help available online (for example, Beat, the UK's eating disorder charity, has lots of information and support, and runs a helpline, and the Government of Western Australia's Centre for Clinical Interventions is a great resource for teenagers and their parents), but it is also absolutely okay to seek help in person. You are entitled to seek help no matter how much you weigh or what your body looks like. Asking for help as early as possible to help manage your relationship with food is the best, most proactive course of action. So if you feel like your relationship with food and eating is controlling and taking over your life, go and speak to an adult you trust or visit your GP. Your GP can then refer you to a specialist who will do their best to help you, no matter how big or small the problem. Early intervention leads to the best outcomes.

Eating issues can affect people in lots of ways. For example, you might:

- Find that controlling food or eating has become the most important thing in your life

- Feel depressed, anxious, guilty or ashamed, and scared of other people finding out

- Feel distant from friends or family who don't know how you feel or who are frustrated and upset that they can't do more to help

- Avoid social occasions, dates and restaurants or eating in public

- Find that other people comment on your appearance in ways you find difficult

- Find that you are bullied or teased about food and eating

- Develop short- or long-term physical health problems

- Find that you have to drop out of school or college, or stop doing things you enjoy.

If someone has an eating disorder like anorexia nervosa or bulimia nervosa, it will have an impact on their health and they are likely to display some outward signs of it. In fact, these disorders have a range of physical symptoms.

SYMPTOMS OF AN EATING DISORDER

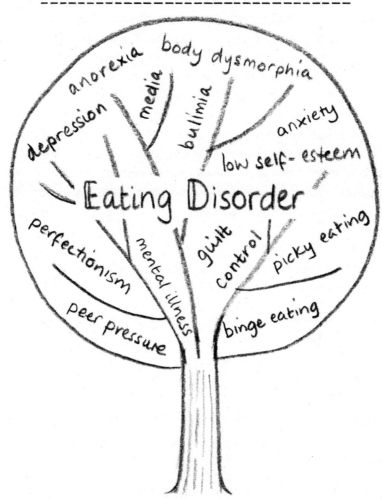

❛ I was struggling with *school. I wanted to do well, but found the day-to-day challenges overwhelming a lot of the time. To offset the stresses of the day I binge-watched YouTube until late into the night and then crawled out of bed in the morning. I'd skip breakfast most days, and then lacked focus and motivation during the day, having naps when I could. The teachers always said they felt I had potential, but I never managed to get good grades. As boring as it sounds, by creating proper mealtimes, eating breakfast and not staying up till way after midnight has made a huge difference. I did really well at my GCSEs and am so happy I made the changes.* **I am much happier with my life now** *I have better eating habits and some routines that work for me.* ❜

BELLA (17)

✳ Summary ✳

There are no bad or good foods and we don't have to eat healthily all the time. The 80:20 rule allows us to eat well 80% of the time and be more relaxed about food for 20% of the time. There are also lots of strategies we can use to **help us control what we eat,** including when we're socialising, and meal plans that incorporate all the important food groups each day and throughout the week are key to this.

Unfortunately, our healthy relationship with food can sometimes break down and an eating disorder is when people stop eating properly. As well as being distressing for the person who has the eating disorder, this can cause problems with growth and development. It can be very hard to ask for help, but if you feel you may have an eating disorder, please **don't feel afraid to talk to an adult you trust** about it. The sooner the issue is addressed, the sooner you will recover.

Chapter 15

Managing your emotions around food

Human beings love to eat for many more reasons than sustenance or to satisfy our hunger. Have you ever reached for a tub of ice cream when you're feeling down? Or ordered a pizza at the end of a long week when you're tired? We often use food for comfort, stress relief or as a reward and when we do we tend towards more unhealthy treat foods or high-sugar and -fat foods.

Emotional eating is using food to make us feel better, to fill our emotional needs, rather than our stomach. So many of us use food to cope with emotions, but if we are lonely, sad or bored, food won't fix any of these feelings. More often than not, emotional eating can make us feel worse, bringing feelings of guilt for overeating, while the initial problem remains unresolved. It may provide a little distraction of deliciousness for the short term or even numb you for a short while, but food won't solve the problem and you'll ultimately have to deal with the source of the emotion.

Are you an emotional eater?

- Do you eat when you feel down?
- Do you eat when you feel anxious?
- Do you eat when you feel stressed?
- Do you eat when you're not actually hungry?
- Do you carry on eating even when you're full?
- Do you eat as a reward to yourself?
- Do you feel unable to control your response to food?

Emotional eating triggers

In order to manage emotional eating, it is important to identify what your personal triggers are. Try to notice what situations, places or feelings make you turn to food for comfort. Although it is more common for emotional eating to be triggered by negative and unpleasant emotions, positive feelings and experiences may also be a trigger, such as rewarding yourself for a goal, celebrating a holiday or a happy event.

THE EMOTIONAL EATING CYCLE

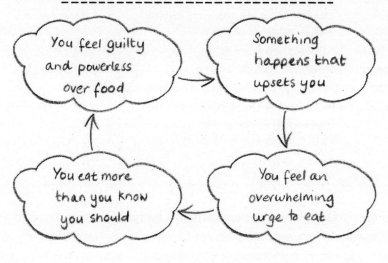

Keep an emotional eating food diary

One of the best ways to identify the patterns behind your emotional eating is to keep track with a food and mood diary.

Every time you feel the urge to overeat or feel the need to reach for your favourite comfort food, take a moment to work out what feeling or situation triggered this. Once you have pinpointed the emotion, write it all down: what you ate, what happened to upset you, how you felt before you ate, what you felt as you were eating and how you felt afterwards.

Food and mood diary example

DAY 3		
Time	Food and drink	Energy levels and mood changes
7.30am	Breakfast: Small tin of beans 2 slices of granary toast	Lots of energy Good mood
9.20am	Tea with milk and sugar	Bit insecure (personal reasons)
11am	Glass of water	Quite stressed, hard to focus
12pm	1 slice of granary toast and butter	
3pm	Glass of water	Not as agitated,
4pm	Lunch: Beef stroganoff with rice 7 chunks of pineapple	but a bit tired
5.30pm	Glass of water	
7pm	Small packet of Doritos	Much calmer
9pm	Dinner: 4 fish fingers, mashed potatoes, peas and sweetcorn. Glass of orange juice Decaf tea with milk and sugar 1 petits filous	Better mood Skin on arms very itchy Good mood Tired
10.30pm	Glass of water	

Over time you might see patterns emerge. Perhaps you feel the need to eat after spending time with a particular friend who may be critical of you? Or maybe you stress-eat whenever you're on a deadline or when you attend family functions. As soon as you identify what your personal triggers are, the next step is to find healthier ways to feed those feelings.

How to tell the difference between physical and emotional hunger

Physical hunger...	Emotional hunger...
Comes on slowly and gradually	Arrives out of nowhere
Is pretty easy to ignore for a while	Feels urgent
Can be satisfied with pretty much whatever's on offer	Is very specific about what will satisfy it
Goes away when you're full	Doesn't really go away
Doesn't set off bad feelings	Triggers powerful feelings, making you feel, for example, worthless or guilty

Change the story in your head

We all talk to ourselves all day long, a little voice that never seems to shut up, and what that inner voice says is important. Perhaps the voice constantly self-criticises, misinterprets or overanalyses situations. If so, try changing your internal dialogue to more empowering thoughts and messages: 'I'm really proud of myself for saying no to unhealthy snacks – I make conscious choices to look after myself and choose healthy snacks and treats' or 'I will reward myself with a healthy treat when I've achieved my exam result'. How about changing the reward to a trip to the cinema, going ice skating or having your nails done?

Create other ways to feed your feelings

To manage emotional eating, it's important to find other ways to fulfil yourself emotionally. It is vital to understand and know your triggers, but that's just the first step. You will need to find replacements for food, so that you can fill your emotional needs in healthier and more satisfying ways. Here are some ways to replace emotional eating:

- If you're depressed or lonely, call someone who always makes you feel better, play with your dog or cat, maybe watch a feel-good movie, lift your mood by playing happy music or offer to volunteer at a local charity

- If you're anxious, expend your nervous energy by dancing to your favourite music, take a brisk walk, go for a jog or try deep breathing techniques (see pages 160–161)

- If you're exhausted, treat yourself with a hot cup of tea, take a bath, light some scented candles, wrap yourself in a warm blanket, read a good book and get an early night

- If you're bored, learn to cook a new recipe, read a good book, watch a comedy show, go outside and exercise or turn to an activity you enjoy – playing the guitar, drawing, cooking, yoga

Eat mindfully

Emotional eating often happens so quickly and mindlessly that you miss out on the different tastes and textures of your food. Not only this, but you also miss your body's cues that tell you when you are full. To stop this, try to slow down and savour every bite. By taking the time to do this you'll enjoy your food more and also be less likely to overeat.

Slowing down the process and savouring your food is a crucial aspect of eating mindfully. Take a few deep breaths before starting your food. Put your utensils down between bites and really focus on the experience of eating. Enjoy it! Pay attention to the textures, shapes, colours and smells of your food. How does each mouthful taste? How does it make your body feel? Note these positive experiences in your food and mood diary too.

By generally eating more slowly, you'll find you're satisfied by smaller amounts of food and, because it takes time for the message that you're full to reach your brain, taking a few moments to consider how you feel after each bite – hungry or satiated – can help you avoid overeating.

Take five before you give in to a craving

Emotional eating is often an automatic or mindless act. You experience your triggers and then, before you even realise it, you've reached for a tub of ice cream and you're three-quarters of the way through it! But if you take a moment to pause and reflect when you're hit with a craving, you give yourself the chance to make a different decision.

Don't dig in that spoon just yet. Can you wait five minutes? Or even one minute? Postponing the moment when you start eating is better than lecturing yourself about how you mustn't give in to the craving, because if you do you'll feel you've failed, plus what's forbidden is always tempting!

And as you wait, take the chance to see how you're feeling? What was it that made you pick up the spoon? What emotions are you experiencing? You may end up eating the ice cream, but if you do at least you'll have a clearer idea of what prompted you to do it and that will be helpful next time.

Try the 5 x 5 approach

We all feel a range of emotions every day, but eating to suppress these feelings can cause us harm in the long term. Learn to recognise your emotions and identify if you are using food because you are bored, sad, fed up or uncomfortable with the emotions that you are feeling.

Here's a useful technique to use when you don't know where to turn. When you're feeling calm and relaxed, use the points below to make five lists of five things. Write them down or note them on your phone, but keep them somewhere you can refer back to when you're feeling overwhelmed. They will act as useful prompts to help you work out what to do next.

- 5 x people you can speak to

- 5 x ways to relax

- 5 x things to say to yourself when you're stressed

- 5 x places that are calming

- 5 x activities that distract you when you feel down

Intuitive eating

Intuitive eating means exactly that – using your intuition to make you the expert on your body, your nutrient requirements and your personal hunger signals. The idea is that you should eat when you're hungry, stop when you're full, and eat the foods your body tells you to and that you enjoy. For example, if you crave iron-rich foods, your body is telling you it needs more iron.

To eat intuitively, you need a certain level of nutritional knowledge about why certain foods lead us to crave them more, you need to be able to distinguish between emotional and physical hunger (see above) and then you need to learn to trust your body.

Don't deliberately deprive yourself of a certain food, because you'll only crave it even more. That craving will build and build until you can't control it. Eventually you'll crack and eat what you crave, but this may make you feel extremely guilty, which may then lead to self-loathing and overeating. If you dial it down and don't ban the food, your emotions will be less intense and perhaps more manageable.

By giving yourself the freedom to eat intuitively, you don't have to live with fear around foods and you give yourself <u>unconditional permission to eat</u>.

So many people develop an unhealthy relationship with food, monitoring every calorie they consume or rewarding themselves because they didn't eat cake. Intuitive eating challenges where those ideas come from and allows you to 'shout them down' and move forward to enjoy all foods, eating to feel good, and optimise your energy and well-being.

In Japanese culture, finding and enjoying 'pleasure' is one of the goals for healthy living. Pleasure is one of the most basic gifts of existence. When we eat what we want and enjoy the food we are eating, we will naturally feel satisfied and content. We can regulate our appetite far better when we enjoy our food than if we obsess over what we should or shouldn't be eating.

✳ Summary ✳

Emotional eating is normal. Having other coping mechanisms, such as adopting the 5 x 5 approach to managing your emotions (see page 155), can help you gain control over emotional eating for good. Learning self-acceptance and developing a positive and pleasurable relationship with food makes for an easier and more contented life. Intuitive eating is simply a way of eating that promotes listening to your body and having a healthy attitude towards food.

Chapter 16

All about anxiety

Anxiety is something most of us have experienced. A difficult conversation with a friend or parent, an exam, an audition for the school play or an interview for a Saturday job – these are things that can cause even the calmest person to feel a little stressed. And that's normal. Figuring out how to deal with that panic is the key.

Everyone feels anxious at times. This is because feeling anxious is part of the body's 'fight or flight' response, preparing you to act quickly in the face of danger – it's how we survived when big scary woolly mammoths were jumping out of bushes at us! But even though life for most of us is less dangerous, this fight or flight response remains. And many things in our daily lives can trigger this response, even though we don't really need to actually physically run away – things like feeling unprepared, waiting for the results of a test or going on a first date.

This five-step exercise can be very helpful during periods of anxiety, because it grounds you in the present when your mind is bouncing around between various anxious thoughts. I use it all the time. Go through the following steps:

- Identify **five** things you can see – it could be your phone, a poster on the ceiling, anything in your immediate environment

- Identify **four** things you can touch – it could be your own hair, the back of a chair or the ground under your feet

- Identify **three** things you can hear – if your tummy is rumbling that counts, but try to focus on things beyond your body

- Identify **two** things you can smell – it could be soap on your hands or something in the natural world if you're outside

- Identify **one** thing you can taste – what does the inside of your mouth taste like?

When anxiety becomes a problem

If the feelings of anxiety become severe or persistent to the point that they interfere with your daily life, then it's important to try to address them. If you have constant feelings of worry, fear and panic, and also experience physical symptoms such as a faster heart rate, breathlessness, nausea, sweating, shaking and an upset tummy, you should aim to use the tools in this chapter to help you overcome the anxiety. It might also be helpful to speak to a healthcare professional.

There's lots of talk about depression, but what about anxiety? Mental health conversations have – until fairly recently – tended to focus on depression, but anxiety disorders are common across all population groups, including young people. Perhaps this rise in anxiety is a result of our fast-paced 21st-century lives or the expectations that have mounted alongside developments in technology and social media?

Stress steals magnesium and B vitamins

Magnesium is an essential mineral that helps us manage our stress levels and our body to function properly. Sleep patterns are often disrupted in individuals with heightened anxiety and a 2001 study found optimal magnesium to be necessary for normal sleep regulation too.

However, anxiety and stress can easily deplete the body's stores. Stress can increase the amount of magnesium we lose through our urine, leading to deficiencies. This creates a vicious cycle whereby we are stressed, we lose more magnesium and the low magnesium leads us to feel more stressed – and on and on.

One of the easiest ways to help us manage stress is to increase our magnesium intake. Many of the whole grains, dark green leafy veg, legumes, and nuts and seeds I encourage you to eat throughout this book are also good sources of magnesium, as are chicken, beef and fatty fish, like mackerel, salmon and halibut. I would point you to bananas, figs, avocados and tofu too.

Magnesium is also absorbed well through the skin. Chemists sell a spray that you rub into your tummy or inner thighs at any time of the day, or increase your magnesium intake with an Epsom salts bath (see page 125).

Stress also depletes our B vitamins and studies show B vitamins help reduce our stress levels, so it's important to ensure you're getting plenty of B vitamins to help manage stress and anxiety, and stabilise your mood. Some of the best sources of B vitamins are red meat (particularly liver, although admittedly it's not to everyone's taste!), chicken, seafood, eggs, dairy products, leafy greens, whole grains, legumes and seeds, as well as fortified foods, like some breakfast cereals and nutritional yeast.

Consider meditation, mindfulness and yoga

Research has shown that just a few minutes of daily meditation practice that includes deep rhythmic breathing can reduce stress and anxiety, and help clear the mind.

If you're a meditation beginner, when you're feeling anxious, close your eyes and breathe in deeply for a count of four, allowing the air to fill your tummy. Hold that breath for a count of four and then breathe out slowly for another count of four. As you breathe, try to visualise a healing white or blue light washing over your body. Over time it's likely you will notice a sense of calm and tranquillity in your mind and body, but it does take practice! Start with a few minutes a day and you can steadily work up to 20 minutes. There are lots of apps and YouTube tutorials out there where you can learn beginner's yoga moves and pranayama (yoga) breathing, which also induces a sense of calm.

Stop scrolling and get active – exercising can really boost our endorphins and our feel-good hormones.

FINDING SOME HEADSPACE

Life can sometimes feel hectic and stressed, and filled with classes and exams, so relaxing and having downtime is essential to staying healthy. Stress can cause lots of problems and getting too run-down can have a negative effect on your health.

The easiest way to make sure you relax is to create a routine and give yourself regular breaks. Make time to hang out with your friends and carve out time to de-stress by reading a book, watching your favourite TV show or picking up a hobby.

If you've never tried it, meditation, and meditation apps like the free Insight app, can help create 'mini vacations' for your racing mind throughout the day. Meditating will enable you to recharge your batteries by reducing the amount of cortisol (the stress hormone) circulating in your body. This will in turn build your resilience and strengthen your long-term immunity.

Just move!

We know that spending time in natural environments, like parks or woodlands or by lakes, can reduce stress, and we know that exercise reduces anxiety too, so try to combine the two if you can.

The key is to find at least one physical activity that you enjoy to help you get your daily dose of fitness in. It could be anything, from dancing, skateboarding, boxing or horse riding to going for a run or to the gym. It doesn't matter what you do, as long as you move.

The big benefits of exercise

Not only does exercise tone your body, it strengthens your muscles, keeps your bones strong and improves your skin. And there are more benefits of exercise – including increased relaxation, better sleep and mood and strong immune function.

Exercise for mental health

Exercise encourages the body's production of endorphins, the chemicals that improve mood. It reduces the risk of depression, increases self-esteem, builds self-confidence and promotes restful sleep.

It also enhances thinking and learning skills, and may improve school performance. This is because the increased blood flow to the brain means the brain receives the oxygen and nutrients it needs promptly and is therefore at the top of its game.

Regular exercise can also be an excellent antidote to stress, because it reduces levels of the stress hormone, which results in lower blood pressure, a slower heart rate and reduced muscle tension, all of which makes you feel calmer.

Exercise for physical health

By boosting your circulation, exercise supports your body's natural detox process and the increased blood flow makes your skin glow. Exercise also gets oxygen to the skin, increasing the production of collagen, which plumps your complexion.

Exercise comes in many forms and is a <u>miracle cure</u> for so many things. Students who exercise vigorously for 20 minutes a day, seven days a week, have been shown to achieve <u>higher grades</u> than students who don't.

Studies show that strengthening exercises, like weight training, builds bone mass and muscle strength, and the more muscle mass you have, the more calories your body burns, even when you're not actually exercising. However, regular, moderate exercise, like walking, jogging, running and dancing, helps your bones stay healthy, too.

And talking of health, exercise appears to reduce the number of colds and other minor illnesses you catch (it gives the immune system a nudge), although if you over-exercise it can have the opposite effect and make you more susceptible to viruses, so do take rest days and always listen to your body.

Get started with exercise

In time you will find exactly the right exercise routine for you, but make sure you include these three types of exercise, if not every day then at least a couple of times in the week:

- Stretching exercises, like yoga or a set of stretches using all parts of the body in sequence, keep your muscles flexible and improve your range of movement.

- Endurance exercises, like walking, cycling, swimming or aerobics, keep your heart and lungs healthy and strengthen your muscles.

- Strengthening exercises, like weight training with free weights or resistance bands, build your muscles.

DON'T FORGET TO HYDRATE

The more intense the training session, the more heat your body will produce. Before beginning any exercise, drink water to help the body compensate for sweating. You can drink more water during the exercise if you're thirsty.

Stress survival guide

Here it is – these are the key actions that will keep you calm and get you through.

Body	Mind	Soul
Healthy sleep	Talk about what's stressing you out	Engage in positive self-talk
Move your body	Keep a stress journal	Practise saying 'no' more
Up your nutrients	Prioritise your time – write lists	Take a break from social media
Deep breathing	Break big tasks into smaller steps	Accept that stress is a normal part of life
Listen to calming music	Set healthy habits and rituals	Try mindfulness
Take a bath	Ask for some help	Let yourself rest if you're feeling overwhelmed – mental health comes first
5–10 minutes of daily meditation	Consider seeing a counsellor if it becomes too much for you	

✳ Summary ✳

When we are undergoing periods of stress or anxiety, it's important we increase our intake of magnesium and B vitamins. Deep breathing, meditation and yoga can also help stop a racing mind, and reduce stress and anxiety. Exercise naturally produces feel-good hormones or endorphins and therefore lifts our mood and energy levels, and spending time in natural environments has been shown to reduce stress hormones too, as has being with friends and family.

Chapter 17

Learning to love yourself

Here is some self-care advice to help you develop a healthy relationship with your body:

- Learn self-acceptance. We are all born totally unique and beautiful in our own way. Please don't waste a moment's energy on wanting to be a different person; work on being the very best version of yourself.

- Stop comparing yourself to others. Wishing you were taller or had curly hair, a different eye colour or a different body shape is all wasted energy. Enjoy who you are and what you look like, and you will find life much more enjoyable.

- Appreciate your uniqueness. You are totally, wonderfully unique (unless you're an identical twin, but even then, there will be many differences in your personality, preferences and so on). Embrace that uniqueness and who you are, starting today!

- Appreciate what your body does for you, not just what it looks like. Your body is an extraordinary machine that undertakes thousands of tasks each day. Respect, appreciate and be in awe of your body, and love it for all it does for you.

- We all have a nagging negative voice in our heads – you know the one I mean – that tells us we aren't good enough. Recognise that voice and practise telling it, 'Actually, I'm enough just as I am.'

Challenge negative thinking

In 2005, the US Government's National Science Foundation published an article that concluded the average person has somewhere between 12,000 and 60,000 thoughts every day. Actually, the exact figure doesn't really matter, but what does matter is that it's very easy for the majority of them to be negative. However, you can nip negative self-talk in the bud and flip to more positive thoughts by being conscious that you are responsible for your thought patterns, and you can challenge – 'nip and flip' – all negative and unhelpful thinking. Here are some prompts to get you started:

POSITIVE PROMPTS

- I am unique because...

- At school I am good at...

- One of my best qualities is...

- My friends like me because...

- My family are proud of me because...

- I am pleased with myself for...

- I am happy when...

- Today I am grateful for...

- I really enjoy...

> 6 **I hated being so tall** and big-framed. It made me
> so sad and upset, and I constantly compared myself
> to my tiny, skinny friends. After attending one of Tina's
> workshops, I started to be kinder to myself. She showed
> us there are so many different body shapes and that we
> are all totally different and unique. We can choose to
> accept and love ourselves or have a lifetime of hatred and
> low self-esteem. **I practise daily gratitude** and do
> the simplest things to care for and respect my body and
> to make me feel good. I focus on how amazing my body
> is and all it does for me, and I make a conscious effort
> to choose much better thoughts. 9

EVE (15)

Look after yourself

Be kind to yourself and learn self-compassion. This is the biggest gift you can give to yourself in your life. Treat yourself like you would your best friend. Don't be tough or scold yourself if you're having a tough time. Be kind and nurturing to yourself.

Learn to create healthy habits that make you feel good about yourself, for example listening to music and dancing in your bedroom, going skateboarding in the park, or doing some yoga or meditation – just find activities that make you feel happy.

You might find the daily and weekly habits checklists on the following pages useful – add in any other good habits that are important to you:

Daily habits checklist	Day 1	Day 2	Day 3	Day 4	Day 5	Day 6	Day 7
Pack my snacks for the day							
Eat a balanced breakfast or make a smoothie to go							
Take time to relax before bed – turn screens off at least an hour before bed or just read a book							
Eat a rainbow of colourful fruits and veggies							
Eat a small handful of mixed unsalted nuts and seeds							
Say at least two positive things about myself							
Follow my fitness plan							
Always walk the long way							
Spend just five minutes breathing deeply to create a sense of calm and tran-quillity							
Smile often – when we smile, it makes other people smile too							

Weekly habits checklist	Week 1	Week 2	Week 3	Week 4
Make a meal plan				
Try at least one new recipe				
Aim to eat at least 30 different plants every week (fruit, veg, beans, legumes, nuts, seeds, herbs, grains – they all count)				
Write out my big-picture and day-to-day goals				
Track my progress and share your accomplishments with others				

Learn self-soothing techniques for when you feel down or sad. Many people use food for comfort and that is absolutely fine, but it shouldn't be the only tool in your toolbox for dealing with stress. We need a range of coping strategies for when we are having a difficult time – for instance, try the 5 x 5 approach, which is a useful technique if you're feeling stressed or sad (see page 155). Create a self-care journal and know what strategies help you to manage your emotions.

How to increase your self-worth

- Be responsible for yourself
- Realise you have control of your thoughts and behaviours
- Choose to think better and more positive thoughts
- Cheer for yourself when you have done something well and recognise what you're good at

- Be nurturing and loving to yourself and your body
- Create healthy habits that allow your body and mind to thrive
- Never compare yourself to others
- Ditch social media if it creates negative feelings in you
- Realise you have total control of your destiny and your future
- Create a daily gratitude journal – write down three things you are grateful for each day

Appreciate your body. Instead of focusing on what you don't like about your body, take time to appreciate what you do like and <u>everything it does for you</u> every day.

Changing your habits – old you, new you!

This book is packed with ideas for small changes you can make that will give you more energy and help you feel healthier, but how do you make sure you stick to those changes? To make any change become a habit it's helpful to create SMART goals, which are:

Specific	Measurable	Attainable	Relevant	Time-based
S	M	A	R	T
Exactly what is it you want to do?	How will you know when you've done it?	Is it something it's possible for you to achieve?	Is it realistic for you to achieve it?	What timeframe do you want to achieve it in?

Try setting some SMART goals to help you achieve your goals for your health and happiness, at school or college or in any area of your life. Here are some examples of SMART goals and you can fill in your own goals below.

	Simple goal	SMART goal
Specific: define your goal clearly so that anyone can understand it	I want to improve my health	By eating five portions of fruit and vegetables every day starting today
Measurable: add some measurements, so you know when you've achieved your goal	I want to start running	I will run 5k by 30 November this year using a Couch to 5k app, starting this week
Attainable: your goal must challenge you, but also be realistic	I want to eliminate sugary drinks from my diet	I will start to cut my sugary drinks down to once a week, starting this week
Relevant: make sure your goals are consistent and relate to your long-term goals	I want to change my lifestyle	I will improve my lifestyle by making conscious food decisions at every meal while focusing on protein, vegetables and healthy fats, starting this week
Time-based: create a timeframe in which you want to accomplish your goal	I want to be healthier	I will set aside 30 minutes a day for exercise and see how I feel after 30 days, starting this week

Intention	Specific	Measurable	Attainable	Relevant	Time-based
What do you want to achieve?	Who? What? Why? Where? When?	How often? How much? How many?	Achievable?	Is it relevant to your ultimate vision?	When?

Self-care checklist

As a reminder to look after yourself physically as well as mentally and emotionally, here's a quick daily self-care checklist:

- ☐ Be kind to myself
- ☐ Shower and brush my teeth
- ☐ Stay hydrated – drink 2 litres of water a day
- ☐ Be active for 20–30 minutes
- ☐ Go outside
- ☐ Take time to do something I enjoy
- ☐ Choose a goal to focus on
- ☐ Challenge all negative thoughts
- ☐ Practise breathing techniques
- ☐ Practise mindfulness
- ☐ Keep an eye on my bowel habits
- ☐ Say something nice to myself every day

✳ Summary ✳

To feel great, you need to eat well, which means a healthy, balanced diet. Challenge any negative thinking and learn to accept yourself as you are. That doesn't mean you can't change, but if you do want to improve your life it helps to set SMART – specific, measurable, attainable, relevant and time-based – goals. Above all, find what makes you happy and be kind to yourself.

You are a beautiful, unique, amazing individual with the potential to do great things with your life. You are the future and my dream for you is to be strong in body and mind, to live your life to its fullest, to enjoy a fulfilling career and have lots of adventures along the way. Taking care of your body is the best thing you can ever do for yourself, and if you create healthy habits your body will reward you!

Quick and easy recipes

Learn new skills in the kitchen with these colourful, nutritious and above all quick and easy recipes for every time of the day. Each vibrant recipe includes nutrition tips and at the end of this section there are some bonus sweet treats.

BREAKFAST

LUNCH OR DINNER

LIGHT MEALS AND QUICK SNACKS

SMOOTHIES

SWEET TREATS

Breakfast

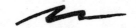

CACAO AND PEANUT BUTTER OVERNIGHT OATS

TINA SAYS

→ If you won't have time to prep in the morning and want to take something with you, just pop the mixture into a glass jar before you put it in the fridge. Chia seeds help to thicken the recipe and are also a great source of fibre and essential fatty acids. Cacao is the unrefined, un-sugared, dried cocoa bean and it's high in magnesium, an important mineral for mood, energy and heart health. ←

Serves 1 ● Prep time: 5 mins

120g porridge oats

375ml almond milk

2 tbsp unsweetened peanut butter

1 tbsp chia seeds

1 banana, mashed, or 1 apple, grated

1 tsp cacao powder

Pinch of sea salt

- In a bowl, mix all the ingredients together well.

- Place the bowl in the fridge overnight, where the mix will thicken, ready to be enjoyed in the morning.

BERRY SMOOTHIE BOWL

Serves 1 • Prep time: 5 mins

4 strawberries, tops cut off

Small handful of blueberries

1 banana, peeled

Flesh of half an avocado

1 heaped tbsp nut butter (e.g. almond)

100ml milk of choice (e.g. cow's, coconut, almond)

1 tbsp chia seeds

A drizzle of nut butter, oats, mixed seeds, chopped fruit and/or a dollop of natural or Greek yoghurt to serve (optional)

- Place the fruit and avocado in a blender with the nut butter, milk and chia seeds, and blend until smooth.

- Transfer the smoothie mixture to a bowl and serve with your choice of toppings.

SHAKSHUKA

Serves 4 • Prep time: 10 mins • Cook time: 15 mins

3 tbsp olive oil

2 large onions, sliced

2 green peppers, sliced

2 red peppers, sliced

4 garlic cloves, crushed

½ tsp cumin seeds

½ tsp ground cumin

½ tsp smoked paprika

1 tbsp tomato purée

2 x 400g tinned tomatoes

8 free-range eggs

85g feta, crumbled

Small bunch fresh parsley, chopped

Salt and pepper, to taste

Sourdough bread or baguette (to serve)

- Heat the olive oil in a large, lidded frying pan. Add the sliced onions and peppers, and cook on a medium heat until softened.

- Add the garlic, both types of cumin and smoked paprika, and cook for a further 2 minutes.

- Stir in the tomato purée and cook for a further 2 minutes, then add the tomatoes with a splash of water (use this to rinse out the tins).

- Simmer for 10 minutes, uncovered. Keep an eye on the texture – it should reduce a little but shouldn't get too dry – and add more water if needed.

- Make eight wells in the sauce, break an egg and drop it in carefully, repeat with each egg.

- Cook until the whites are set, but the yolks are still runny.

- Sprinkle over the crumbled feta and parsley, and season with salt and pepper.

- Serve with sourdough bread or a baguette.

BANANA AND CINNAMON PANCAKES

Serves 2 • Prep time: 10 mins • Cook time: 5 mins

1 egg, beaten

2 tbsp ground flaxseed

1 banana, mashed

1 tsp ground cinnamon

1 tbsp coconut flour or almond flour

1 tbsp plain flour (buckwheat is a gluten-free alternative)

1 tsp baking powder

30–40ml milk of choice

2 tbsp coconut oil

1 tbsp maple syrup

Optional toppings: nut butter, chopped nuts, flaxseeds, chopped or stewed apple

- Place the egg, flaxseed, banana, cinnamon, both flours and the baking powder in a bowl.

- Add the milk and combine the ingredients to make a batter. For American-style pancakes you want a thicker consistency that can be 'dropped' into the pan. Add a further 20–30ml of milk for thinner pancakes.

- Melt the coconut oil in a large frying pan over a medium heat. When hot, pour in 2 tbsp of the pancake batter to make two pancakes.

- Fry the pancakes for 1–2 minutes on each side and flip. They should be lightly browned.

- Stack the warm pancakes on a plate. Drizzle with the maple syrup. If desired, add nut butter, chopped nuts, extra flaxseed, and chopped or stewed apple.

SMASHED AVOCADO AND EGG ON TOAST

Serves 1 • Prep time: 10 mins

1 slice of bread, toasted

½ ripe medium avocado

Small wedge of fresh lemon

1 egg, boiled for 10–12 minutes

Drizzle of extra virgin olive oil

Salt and pepper, to taste

½ handful of fresh parsley, chopped

Small handful of chopped nuts and whole seeds (optional)

- Use a fork to smash the avocado down onto the toasted bread slice.

- Lightly squeeze a small wedge of fresh lemon over the avocado toast.

- Slice the hard-boiled egg in half or into coin shapes and place on top of the smashed avocado.

- Drizzle over the olive oil, season with salt and pepper and sprinkle with the fresh parsley and the nuts and seeds, if desired.

EGG MUFFINS

Makes 10 • Prep time: 10 mins • Cook time: 25 mins

10 eggs

1 courgette, grated

Large handful of spinach, chopped

75g cheese, grated (mozzarella, Cheddar, feta)

4 spring onions, finely sliced

Small handful of fresh chives, chopped

Salt and pepper, to taste

A little olive oil or butter for greasing

Green salad, or a slice of sourdough toast and hummus (to serve)

You will also need a 12-hole muffin tin

- Preheat the oven to 180°C (fan 160°C).

- Crack the eggs into a large bowl and whisk. Add the other ingredients and give the mix a good stir.

- Grease the muffin tin with the oil or butter and spoon equal amounts of the egg mixture into ten of the muffin tin holes. Try to ensure the mixture is distributed as evenly as possible.

- Carefully slide the tin into the oven and bake for around 25 minutes, until the muffins are fully cooked through and lightly golden on top.

- Let them cool for a few minutes before trying to take them out of the tin or they will get stuck.

- Serve with a green salad, or slice of sourdough toast and a dollop of hummus.

COCONUT AND VANILLA OVERNIGHT OATS

→ Full of gut-loving fibre, overnight oats are the ultimate quick breakfast option! ←

Serves 1 • Prep time: 5 mins

120g rolled porridge oats

1 tbsp chia seeds

2 tbsp dessicated coconut

1 tsp cinnamon

2 drops vanilla extract

375ml unsweetened vanilla almond milk

1–2 tbsp frozen berries

Fresh fruit and granola (to serve)

- Place all the ingredients in a bowl or jar.

- Stir to combine and place in the fridge to soak overnight.

- If the mixture is too thick, add some more milk or yoghurt, and serve topped with fresh fruit and granola.

Lunch or dinner

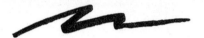

CHICKEN AND BEAN BURRITO

Serves 4 • Prep time: 10 mins • Cook time: 15 mins

4 skinless, boneless chicken thighs

3 tsp smoked paprika

½ tbsp ground cumin

1 tsp chilli flakes

Good drizzle plus 1 tbsp of olive oil

Salt and pepper, to taste

2 garlic cloves, finely sliced

Handful of fresh coriander, leaves roughly chopped, stalks finely sliced

400g tin of black beans

4 large flour tortillas

1 red onion, finely sliced

1 little gem lettuce, shredded

80g mature Cheddar cheese

4 tbsp Greek yoghurt

- Preheat a griddle pan over a high heat. Place the chicken thighs in a bowl, sprinkle over the paprika, cumin, chilli flakes and a good drizzle of olive oil. Season well with sea salt and freshly ground black pepper. Mix well to coat.

- Place the chicken on the hot griddle. Cook for 10 minutes or until charred and cooked through, turning halfway. Leave to cool slightly.

- Heat 1 tbsp of olive oil in a large frying pan over a medium-high heat. Add the garlic and coriander stalks (not leaves) and fry for 1 minute.

- Drain, rinse and add the beans, then fry for a further few minutes. Add the coriander leaves.

- Shred the lettuce and cooled chicken.

- Pop a tortilla onto the griddle for 1 minute to soften it, then place it on a plate. Spoon one-quarter of the fried beans along the middle, top with some red onion, a handful of lettuce and one of the shredded chicken thighs. Grate over some cheese and add a tablespoon of yoghurt. Wrap up the burrito, then tuck in the ends.

- Repeat with the remaining ingredients, serving as you go.

VEGGIE BOWL

Serves 1 • Prep time: 10 mins • Cook time: 30 mins

2 tbsp olive oil

1 sweet potato, cubed

1 tbsp smoked paprika

400g chickpeas, drained and rinsed

1 tsp ground cumin

Pinch of sea salt

½ pack of pre-cooked quinoa

¼ red cabbage, finely sliced

Large handful of rocket or spinach

1 heaped tbsp hummus

Small handful of mixed seeds

- Preheat the oven to 200°C.

- To make the smoky paprika sweet potato, place the potato cubes onto a baking tray and coat with half the olive oil and the smoked paprika. Roast for 25–30 minutes until they begin to brown and soften.

- To make the crispy chickpeas, heat the remaining oil in a frying pan over a medium heat, then add the chickpeas, cumin and a pinch of sea salt. Fry for 90 seconds until golden brown, stirring throughout.

- To build the veggie bowl, put the cooked quinoa in one side of a large bowl, add the roasted sweet potato cubes, crispy chickpeas, finely sliced red cabbage and spinach/rocket, and dollop the hummus on top. Sprinkle with the seeds.

MISO SALMON NOODLES

Serves 2 • Prep time: 15 mins • Cook time: 10 mins

2 tbsp miso paste

750ml boiling water

2 tbsp soy sauce

100g dried egg noodles

1 tbsp coconut oil

1 small aubergine, cubed

1 thumb-print size piece of fresh ginger, peeled and grated

50g cashews

2 pak choi

2 spring onions

2 garlic cloves, finely sliced

1 red chilli, deseeded and finely sliced

Tin of salmon, drained

Handful of fresh coriander, roughly chopped

1 tsp sesame seeds

Salt and pepper, to taste

- Put the miso paste and boiling water in a glass measuring jug.

- Add the soy sauce and stir well, making a broth. Add the dried noodles and set aside.

- Heat the coconut oil in a large wok or wide saucepan. Stir-fry the cubed aubergine, ginger and cashews for roughly 3 minutes, until lightly browned.

- Add the pak choi, spring onions, garlic, chilli and drained salmon, and cook for 2 minutes.

- Add the stock and noodles, separating the noodles with a fork. Allow to simmer for 2 minutes until the noodles are tender.

- Sprinkle with coriander and sesame seeds, and season with salt and pepper.

BUILD YOUR OWN OPEN SANDWICH

→ This is a super speedy lunch and if you choose the
required number of options from each list it will
be nutritious and well balanced. ←

Serves 1

Wholegrain or sourdough bread

Protein options	Leafy green options	Colourful topper options
Tuna	Pea shoots	Sliced tomatoes
Mackerel pâté	Rocket	Sun-dried tomatoes
Cottage cheese	Baby spinach	Artichokes
Hummus	Fresh herbs	Olives
Bean dip	Watercress	Capers
Meat pâté	Romaine lettuce	Cucumber, sliced
Boiled egg	Collard greens	Radishes, sliced
Cheese, sliced	Mustard greens	
Nut butter		

- Take one or two slices of bread. Toast them if desired.
- Select one option from the protein list, one or two options from the leafy green list and two or three options from the colourful toppers list.
- Layer on the bread to create a colourful, nutritious open sandwich.

MEXICAN QUINOA SOUP

Serves 4 • Prep time: 10 mins • Cook time: 40 mins

1 onion, peeled and diced

3 garlic cloves, minced

2 tsp ground cumin

1 tbsp olive oil

400g chopped tinned tomatoes

1 litre vegetable stock

180g quinoa, dried

1 red pepper, deseeded and sliced

Juice of 1 lime, freshly squeezed

½ 400g tin of kidney beans, drained and rinsed

½ 400g tin of black beans, drained and rinsed

½ 200g tin of sweetcorn, drained and rinsed

½ tsp dried chilli flakes

Salt and pepper, to taste

Handful of fresh coriander, roughly chopped

Optional toppings: fresh chilli, grated cheese, a wedge of lime and diced avocado

- In a large, deep saucepan, sauté the onions, garlic, and cumin in the olive oil. Make sure the garlic and onion begin to soften, but don't brown.

- Add the tinned tomatoes and gently simmer for 2–3 minutes.

- Add the vegetable stock and quinoa, and stir through. Increase the temperature and bring to the boil.

- Reduce the heat, cover the pan and allow to simmer for approximately 15–20 minutes until the quinoa is tender. If required, add more water.

- Add the red pepper, lime juice, kidney beans, black beans and sweetcorn. Simmer for a further 10–15 minutes.

- Add the chilli flakes, and season with salt and pepper.

- Serve in a bowl, topped with your choice of toppings such as fresh coriander, fresh chilli, grated cheese, a wedge of lime and even try diced avocado. Keep any leftover beans and sweetcorn in the fridge and add them to a Buddha Bowl (see page 201) for a nutritious lunch or dinner.

SUPER GREEN PASTA

Serves 2 • Prep time: 5 mins • Cook time: 15–20 mins

1 tbsp olive oil

1 courgette, sliced

250g fresh spinach

100g frozen peas

2 garlic cloves, crushed

2 portions of wholewheat/green pea/lentil/chickpea pasta

5 cashew nuts

Large handful of fresh basil

Juice of half a lemon

Tin of salmon, drained (optional)

Handful of pine nuts

- In a large pan, heat the olive oil over a medium heat. Add the courgette and sauté for 8–10 minutes until softened and slightly browning.

- Add the spinach, peas and garlic. Cook for a further 3 minutes and then take off the heat.

- Cook the pasta as per the pack instructions.

- While the pasta is cooking, blend the cooked courgette, spinach, peas and garlic, cashews, basil and lemon juice to make a green sauce. If it's too thick, add a little water.

- Drain the pasta, stir in the green sauce.

- Add the salmon if using and heat through for 3–4 minutes, until piping hot.

- Sprinkle with the pine nuts.

STUFFED SWEET POTATO SKINS

TINA SAYS

→ Sweet potatoes are a great source of fibre, vitamins and minerals. However, they are lower in protein, so adding the red kidney beans and cheese increases the protein content to create a balanced meal. ←

Serves 1 • Prep time: 5 mins • Cook time: 30 mins

1 large sweet potato

Pinch of chilli flakes

Small handful of fresh chives, roughly chopped

1½ tbsp olive oil

½ red pepper, deseeded and diced

½ tin red kidney beans, drained

70g cherry tomatoes, quartered

2 spring onions, finely sliced

15g mozzarella, grated or shredded

Lime wedges and guacamole (to serve)

- Preheat the oven to 200°C.

- Pierce the skin of the sweet potato and microwave on a high power for 8–10 minutes until soft.

- Leave the potato to cool slightly, then slice it in half lengthways. Scoop the flesh into a bowl, stir in the chilli flakes and chives, and set aside.

- Put the potato skins on a baking tray in the oven, skin side up, and bake for 8–10 minutes until crisp.

- While they're cooking, heat half of the olive oil in a frying pan. Add the pepper, kidney beans, tomatoes and spring onion. Gently fry for 5 minutes until soft. When cooked, add to the bowl with the sweet potato flesh. Stir through.

- Spoon the filling into the crispy skins and top with the cheese.

- Slide these under a hot grill for 2–3 minutes, until the cheese is melted, and serve with lime wedges and guacamole.

PRAWN LINGUINE

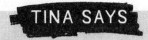
Serves 2 • Prep time: 8 mins • Cook time: 12 mins

160g linguine

½ red onion, diced

2 large garlic cloves, crushed

½ fresh red chilli, deseeded and finely sliced

Handful of cherry tomatoes

Zest of ½ lemon and a squeeze of the juice

1 pack of prawns

Handful of fresh parsley, chopped

- Put the pasta on to cook as per the pack instructions.

- In a large frying pan, sauté the onion, garlic and chilli until softened.

- Add the tomatoes and lightly press them down as they cook. They will burst and split, releasing some juice.

- Add the lemon zest and juice.

- Add the prawns and cook for around 2–4 minutes (or follow pack instructions) until cooked through, but ensuring they don't over-cook (if using frozen prawns, follow the timings on the pack).

- When the pasta is cooked, drain it, reserving a little of the starchy pasta water to add to the sauce.

- Stir the pasta and sauce together and serve in a bowl.

- Sprinkle with the fresh parsley and a squeeze more lemon if desired.

PEANUT AND TOFU STIR-FRY

Serves 1 • Prep time: 10 mins • Cook time: 10 mins

1 tbsp soy sauce

1 tsp rice vinegar

1 tsp maple syrup or honey

1 tsp toasted sesame oil

1 heaped tsp peanut butter

60g egg or rice noodles

150g tofu, cubed

Pinch of salt

¼ tsp chilli flakes

2 tbsp olive oil

1 garlic clove, peeled and sliced

1 carrot, peeled and cut into ribbons or matchsticks

125g broccoli

A handful of coriander, finely chopped

20g roasted peanuts, roughly chopped

- To make the dressing, mix the soy sauce, rice vinegar, maple syrup or honey, sesame oil and peanut butter together in a bowl.

- Cook the noodles as per the pack instructions, then drain and rinse well. Add to the bowl with the dressing.

- Mix the tofu cubes with the salt and the chilli flakes.

- Heat a wok or frying pan over a medium heat, add 1 tbsp olive oil and the tofu, and fry for a couple of minutes until crisp, stirring only occasionally. Put aside on a plate.

- Add the remaining oil to the pan, followed by the garlic, carrot, and broccoli. Cook for around 5 minutes until softened.

- Tip the veg over the noodles, then pile on the tofu and mix together.

- Sprinkle with the coriander and peanuts.

CHICKEN, AVOCADO AND SWEETCORN TACOS

Serves 2 ● Prep time: 15 mins ● Cook time: 15 mins

2 tbsp extra virgin olive oil

1 red onion, diced

4 garlic cloves, peeled and finely chopped

2 chicken breasts or boneless and skinless thighs, diced

2 tbsp tomato purée

½ tsp dried chilli flakes

100g tinned sweetcorn, drained

Flesh of 3 ripe avocados, sliced

4 corn tortillas

½ lime

Handful of coriander or parsley, chopped

Salt and pepper, to taste

- Heat the oil in a saucepan over a medium heat. Add the onion and garlic, cook for a few minutes until softened, and then add the chicken.
- Mix the tomato purée and chilli flakes together, then add them and the sweetcorn to the chicken. Mix through and sauté until the chicken is cooked.
- Build the tacos, adding the chilli corn mix and avocado to the tortillas.
- Add a squeeze of lime, sprinkle with the fresh herbs and season with salt and pepper.

PITTA PIZZA

Serves 1 Prep time: 10 mins • Cook time: 5 mins

Small knob of butter

Handful of baby spinach

1 large round wholemeal pitta or large flatbread

3 tbsp tomato purée

5 black olives, pitted

4–5 cherry tomatoes, halved

1 garlic clove, peeled and sliced

50g feta or mozzarella

Small sprig of fresh basil leaves

Drizzle of olive oil

1 egg (optional)

- Preheat the grill to medium-high.

- Put the butter in a pan and wilt the spinach in it over a medium heat.

- Take the pitta or flatbread and spread the tomato purée over it. Evenly distribute the olives, tomatoes and garlic, spread the cooked spinach over the top and sprinkle with the cheese. If you want to, make a well in the centre of the toppings and crack an egg into it. Drizzle olive oil over the pitta pizza.

- Pop it under the hot grill for around 5 minutes, but keep an eye on it and remove when the edges brown and the egg, if added, is cooked.

BUDDHA BOWL

Serves 1 Prep time: 15 mins

2 tbsp hummus

3 tbsp brown rice or quinoa, cooked and cooled

½ carrot, grated

½ courgette, grated

½ avocado, sliced

2 tbsp tinned kidney beans

handful watercress

2 tbsp tinned sweetcorn

2 radishes, sliced

2 tbsp tahini (sesame paste)

2 tbsp yoghurt

1 garlic clove, crushed

2 tbsp olive oil

Juice of 1 lemon

Salt and pepper, to taste

Sprinkling of pomegranate seeds

- Take a large bowl and spoon the hummus into the centre of it.

- Place the brown rice, carrot, courgette, avocado, beans, watercress, sweetcorn and radishes around the hummus, each in their own separate section.

- Stir the tahini and yoghurt together. Add the remaining ingredients and mix to make a smooth paste, with a few tablespoons of water if needed, then pour the dressing over the contents of the bowl and sprinkle with the pomegranate seeds.

VEGGIE OR PRAWN SATAY NOODLES

Serves 2 Prep time: 15 mins • Cook time: 8 mins

2 tsp sesame oil

1 red onion, finely diced

1 carrot, finely chopped

1 pepper, sliced

1 broccoli head, chopped into small florets

1 garlic clove, finely diced

Thumb-sized piece of ginger, peeled and finely diced

1 small pack of prawns (optional)

200g rice noodles

2 tbsp peanut butter

2 tbsp tamari or soy sauce

Juice of 1 lime

2 tbsp water

Handful fresh coriander (optional)

1 tbsp sesame seeds (optional)

- Heat 1 tsp of sesame oil in a pan, add the onion, carrot, pepper, broccoli, garlic and ginger, and fry for 3 minutes until the vegetables soften. If you're adding prawns, do that now and stir-fry for 3 minutes.

- Cook the rice noodles as per the pack instructions.

- In a small bowl, mix the peanut butter, tamari, the remaining sesame oil, half the lime juice and 1 tbsp water (add more if it's not liquid enough).

- Drain the cooked noodles, add them to the pan with the rest of the lime juice and coriander (if using) and mix. Sprinkle with sesame seeds (if using).

WILD SALMON FISHCAKES

Serves 4 • Prep time: 10 mins • Cook time: 15 mins

800g potatoes, peeled and diced

50ml milk

200g frozen peas

3 spring onions, finely chopped

2 x 145g tins of wild salmon, drained

Salt and pepper, to taste

2 eggs, lightly beaten

200g fresh breadcrumbs

2 tbsp olive oil

Salad or vegetables of choice (to serve)

- Boil the potatoes for 10 to 15 minutes until tender, transfer to a large bowl and mash with the milk.

- Boil the peas for 2 minutes, drain and mix into the mash with the spring onions, salmon, and salt and pepper.

- Shape the mixture into 12 patties. Dip each one in the beaten egg, letting any excess drip off, and then in the breadcrumbs.

- Heat the oil in a non-stick frying pan, add three fishcakes at a time and cook for about three minutes on each side until golden and crispy. Drain these on kitchen paper and then repeat until all the patties are cooked.

- Serve with salad or your favourite vegetables.

Light meals and quick snacks

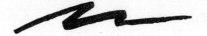

TEN TO THROW TOGETHER WHEN YOU'RE HUNGRY

- **Tuna melt jacket potatoes:** tinned tuna with cheese, spring onions and peas on a microwaved jacket potato

- **Fresh pasta with pesto,** tinned wild salmon and peas

- **Veggie and salad tortilla wraps** with warmed falafel, hummus, shredded red cabbage, salad, beetroot, tomato and coriander

- **Sizzling fajitas:** slice up red onions, peppers, chicken or steak and sauté on a high heat for 5 mins with fajita herbs, then load onto tortilla wraps with extra salad, tomatoes and crushed avocado with coriander

- **Puff pastry pizza:** lay a puff pastry sheet on an oiled baking tray, add tomato pizza topping, mozzarella, anchovies, olives, fresh pesto and basil, and bake in the oven for 25 mins on 200°C

- **Mushroom and spinach tagliatelle:** sauté sliced mushrooms, shredded spinach and chopped garlic, stir into freshly cooked tagliatelle and top with Parmesan shavings

- **Avocado baked eggs:** heat the oven to 220°C, halve a large avocado and remove the stone, put it in a small baking dish, crack an egg into the well left by the stone, sprinkle with paprika, then bake for 15–20 minutes until bubbling

- **Quinoa salad:** add chopped fresh tomatoes, peppers, cucumber, fresh herbs and roasted peppers (from a jar) to ready-to-eat quinoa, and top with unsalted nuts, such as pistachios

- **Lentil and goat's cheese salad:** fry some red onions, garlic, chilli and cumin in a little olive oil, add some pre-cooked Puy lentils and heat through, top with some slices of grilled goat's cheese, sliced sun-dried tomatoes and fresh herbs, and drizzle with vinaigrette dressing

- **Veggie slaw:** mix together a quarter of shredded red and a quarter of shredded white cabbage, a small sliced red onion, two medium grated carrots and two teaspoons of mixed seeds, then stir in a dressing made of two tablespoons of olive oil, one tablespoon of lemon juice, one minced garlic clove, and pinches of cumin and salt. This makes four portions and lasts in the fridge for three days, so you can use as a side dish for any meal or pop into sandwiches or wraps

TEN TOPPINGS FOR WHOLEGRAIN TOAST

- Hummus, cucumber, beetroot and olives

- Cream cheese and frozen berries (defrosted and warmed) with fresh mint

- Tuna, celery, red onions and cucumber, mixed into mayonnaise

- Nut butter (almond, cashew or mixed nut) with bananas

- Avocado, scrambled eggs, cayenne pepper and micro-sprouts

- Cream cheese, smoked salmon, red onions, cucumber and capers

- Tahini, strawberries, cinnamon and honey

- Nut butter, Greek yoghurt, banana, blueberries, strawberries and chia seeds

- Avocado, tomatoes, poached egg and chives

- Speedy mackerel pâté: Skin a pack of smoked mackerel and crush it with a fork in a bowl. Add 2 teaspoons of crème fraîche, a squeeze of lemon juice and fresh black pepper.

Smoothies

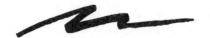

RAINBOW SMOOTHIE

→ This tasty smoothie is a great immune booster. Rich in vitamin A and packed with many minerals to make healthy strong bones and enzymes to help turn our food into energy. ←

Serves 1 • Prep time: 5 mins

1 apple

2 carrots

1 stalk celery

1 handful spinach leaves

1 handful kale

¼ cucumber

2-3cm broccoli stem

1 raw beetroot

¼ courgette

A few fresh mint leaves

2 or 3 ice cubes

- Chop all the ingredients, pop into a blender and blitz until smooth.

- Store any leftovers in a glass bottle in the fridge.

BERRY BLASTER SMOOTHIE

TINA SAYS

→ This berry blaster is packed with so much good stuff and tastes fantastic. The berries help keep your memory sharp and can boost your mood too. The avocado has monounsaturated fats, which keeps your skin plump and smooth. ←

Serves 1 • Prep time: 5 mins

2 handfuls of frozen mixed berries

½ cucumber

¼ lemon

1 pear

1 handful of kale, spinach or any other green leafy veg

½ avocado

2 or 3 ice cubes

- Pop all the ingredients into a blender and pulse until smooth.

- Store any leftovers in a glass bottle in the fridge.

TASTY GREEN SMOOTHIE

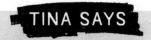

Serves 1 • Prep time: 5 mins

1 frozen banana

1 apple

30g spinach, fresh or frozen

1 tbsp almond butter

150ml coconut water or fresh
apple juice

1–2 fresh mint leaves

Squeeze of lime juice

- Place all the ingredients in a blender.

- Pulse until smooth and pour into a glass to drink.

Sweet treats

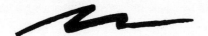

RASPBERRY, ALMOND AND WHITE CHOCOLATE MUFFINS

TINA SAYS

→ These are so much healthier and delicious than shop-bought muffins and take no time at all to throw together. Get into the habit of preparing your own treats and snacks to save money and feel nourished.

Cooking with ground almonds is a great addition to recipes. It's packed with nutrients and slightly sweet, meaning you need less sugar in your recipes. It's a great source of protein, calcium, fibre and healthy fats. ←

Makes 12 • Prep time: 8 mins • Cook time: 25 mins

3 eggs

125ml light and mild olive oil

200ml skimmed milk

3 or 4 drops almond extract

200g self-raising flour

100g golden caster sugar

100g ground almonds

75g white chocolate chips

250g raspberries

75g flaked almonds

- Preheat the oven to 180°C.

- Line a 12-hole muffin tin with paper cases.

- Beat the eggs with the oil, milk and almond extract.

- Place the flour, sugar, ground almonds and chocolate chips in a large bowl.

- Mix the wet ingredients into the dry ingredients until just blended, taking care not to overmix – the mixture should be lumpy. Stir in the raspberries until just mixed with the batter.

- Divide the batter between the paper cases and scatter the flaked almonds on top.

- Bake for 20–25 minutes or until well risen, springy to the touch and golden brown.

EASIEST NO-BAKE ENERGY BALLS

TINA SAYS

→ These are power packed for sustainable energy and a great pick-me-up if you are feeling tired or need to eat before exercise. Try swapping in chopped frozen raspberries to give them a fresh flavour rather than the cinnamon. ←

Makes 15 balls • Prep time: 10 mins

90g porridge oats (not jumbo or rolled oats)

150g peanut butter or almond butter

2 heaped tbsp cocoa powder

3 tbsp honey or maple syrup

2 tbsp chia seeds

1 tsp cinnamon (optional)

Desiccated coconut or ground pistachios (for coating)

- Put all the ingredients except the coconut into a bowl and mix with your hands into a dough, roll into balls and then roll in the coconut, ground pistachios or some additional cocoa powder to finish.

- If you feel that the consistency is too thick, you can add some additional honey or maple syrup.

- Keeps in a sealed container in the fridge for up to two weeks.

FRUITY BREAKFAST LOAF

→ **Buckwheat is a gluten and grain-free flour that has more protein, fibre and B-vitamins than an equal amount of wheat flour, so it's more nutritious. It can help provide stable energy levels too.** ←

Makes 8–12 portions • Prep time: 15 mins • Cook time: 45 mins

2 large or 3 small very ripe bananas

2 eggs or 2 flax eggs (see page 218)

2 tbsp almond milk

1 tsp vanilla extract

4 tbsp coconut oil, melted

4 tbsp honey or maple syrup

200g buckwheat flour

50g oats, plus a spare sprinkle

2 tbsp chopped walnuts or pistachios

1 tsp cinnamon

1 ½ tsp baking powder

½ tsp baking soda

150g fresh raspberries or blueberries

Extra oats, for sprinkling

- Preheat the oven to 180°C.

- Line a loaf tin with grease-proof paper.

- In a large bowl, mash the bananas. Whisk in the eggs or flax eggs, almond milk, vanilla extract, melted coconut oil and honey or maple syrup.

- In another bowl, mix together the flour, oats, nuts, cinnamon, baking powder and baking soda.

- Fold the dry ingredients into the wet and mix well. Stir in the berries.

- Pour into the tin and spread out evenly. Sprinkle the top with some extra oats.

- Bake for 45 minutes.

- Allow to cool in the tin for 10 minutes before turning out and cooling on a rack.

BLACK BEAN BROWNIES

➔ The unexpected black beans in this recipe are super high in fibre, great for our gut bacteria, and they provide a fudgy texture that can compete with traditional flour/sugar brownies. ←

Makes 9–12 brownies • Prep time: 10 mins • Cook time: 18 mins

1 tin black beans, drained and rinsed

3 tbsp cacao powder

80g maple syrup

40g coconut oil, melted

2 tsp vanilla extract

40g fine oats

½ tsp baking powder

115g dark chocolate, broken into small pieces, or chocolate chips

Tiny pinch of sea salt

Walnut pieces or extra chocolate chips, for sprinkling (optional)

- Heat the oven to 175°C.

- Combine all the ingredients other than the chocolate in a food processor.

- Blend until completely smooth.

- Stir in the chocolate and pour into a greased oven tray or pan.

- Sprinkle walnut pieces or extra chocolate chips on the surface.

- Bake for 15–18 minutes. Allow to cool before removing from the tray and cutting. Don't worry if they look a little undercooked – they firm up in the fridge and this gives them a fudgy texture.

BANANA AND CASHEW NICE CREAM

Serves 4 • Prep time: 5 mins • Freezing time: 20 mins

4 frozen bananas, peeled and sliced

60ml cashew, almond, coconut or soy milk

65g cashew butter

Pinch of sea salt

- Place the bananas and milk in a food processor or blender. Blend and pulse until smooth. Don't over-blend, as this will melt the banana.

- Add the cashew butter and pinch of salt and pulse to combine.

- Enjoy immediately as a soft serve or transfer to the freezer in a suitable container. Once frozen solid, it will need to sit at room temperature for around 20 minutes until it softens to a creamier texture for eating.

SUPER-HEALTHY MUFFINS

Makes 6 large or 12 small • Prep time: 10 mins • Cook time: 25 mins

200g spelt flour

2 eggs or 2 flax eggs

1 tsp ground ginger

1 tsp cinnamon

1 tsp baking powder

¾ tsp bicarbonate of soda

170ml light and mild olive oil

225g tin of pineapple in its own juice, crushed

Large carrot, grated

1 courgette, grated

100g of raisins, grated apple or blueberries (optional)

4 tsp honey or maple syrup.

- Preheat the oven to 160°C.

- Mix the ingredients together in a large bowl and pour into muffin cases.

- Bake for 25 minutes.

Further reading and resources

The beginner's guide to a plant-based diet

Bosh! All Plants, Ian Theasby and Henry Firth, HQ (2018)

Deliciously Ella, Ella Woodward, Yellow Kite (2015)

How To Go Plant-Based, Ella Mills, founder of Deliciously Ella, Hodder & Stoughton (2022)

The Medicinal Chef: Plant-based Diet, Dale Pinnock, Hamlyn (2021)

The Plant Power Doctor, Dr Gemma Newman, Ebury Press (2021)

https://www.forksoverknives.com/how-tos/plant-based-primer -beginners-guide-starting-plant-based-diet/#gs.6jh63h

https://www.vegansociety.com/go-vegan

https://vegsoc.org

Intuitive eating

The Doctor's Kitchen, Dr Rupy Aujla, Thornsons (2017)

Eating Mindfully for Teens: A Workbook to Help You Make Healthy Choices, End Emotional Eating, and Feel Great, Susan Albers, New Harbinger (2018)

Eat Yourself Healthy, Dr Megan Rossi, Penguin Life (2019)

Just Eat It, Laura Thompson, Bluebird (2019)

https://www.bda.uk.com/resource/tired-of-diets-use-intuitive-eating -to-break-free-from-food-rules.html

Improve your mental health

Brain Inflamed, Dr Kenneth Bock, Piatkus (2021)

Happy, Fearne Cotton, Orion Spring (2017)

Happy Mind, Happy Life: 10 Simple Ways to Feel Great Every Day, Dr Ranjan Chatterjee, Penguin Life (2022)

How to Grow Up and Feel Amazing: The No-Worries Guide for Boys, Dr Ranj Singh, Wren & Rook (2012)

The Inflamed Mind: A radical new approach to depression, Professor Edward Bullmore, Short Books Ltd (2019)

The Mindfulness Journal for Teens, Jennie Marie Battistin, Rockridge Press (2019)

Positively Teenage: A positively brilliant guide to teenage well-being, Nicola Morgan, Franklin Watts (2018)

Smart Foods for ADHD and Brain Health: How Nutrition Influences Cognitive Function, Behaviour and Mood, Dr Rachel Gow, Jessica Kingsley Publishers (2021)

The Thrive Programme for 8–18 year olds, Rob Kelly, Rob Kelly Publishing (2017)

You Don't Understand Me: The Young Woman's Guide to Life, Tara Porter, Lagom (2022)

Self-esteem

The Little Box of Confidence, Summersdale Publishers (2022)

The Ultimate Self-Esteem Workbook for Teens, Megan MacCutcheon, Althea Press (2019)

Skin health

Radiant: Recipes to heal your skin from within, Hannah Sillitoe, Kyle Books (2017)

Eating disorders

Orthorexia: When Healthy Eating Goes Bad, Renee McGregor, Nourish Books (2017)

https://www.beateatingdisorders.org.uk

https://www.cci.health.wa.gov.au/Resources/Looking-After-Yourself/Disordered-Eating

Sports nutrition for young athletes

Sports Nutrition for Young Adults, Jackie Slomin, Rockridge Press (2020)

The Vegan Athlete's Cookbook, Anita Bean, Bloomsbury Sport (2021)

Meditation and Breathwork
https://insighttimer.com/meditation-app
https://www.breathwrk.com/
iBreathe - Simple guided breathing app

Food scanning
https://www.nhs.uk/healthier-families/food-facts/nhs-food-
    scanner-app/

Healthy cookbooks
Doctor's Kitchen 3-2-1: 3 fruit and veg, 2 servings, 1 pan, Dr Rupy
    Aujla, Thorsons (2010)
Eat Shop Save: 8 Weeks to Better Health, Dale Pinnock, Hamlyn (2019)

Supplement recommendations

General multivitamins and nutrients
Wild Nutrition
Cytoplan

Vegan supplements
Drvegan.com
Myvegan.com
The Vegan Society

Omega-3 fish and algae oils
Bare Biology
Cytoplan
Nordic Naturals Omega (Algae oil)
Wileys

Protein powders
Bulk.com – offers organic powders
TheProteinWorks.com – includes a great range of vegan powders
Formnutrition.com – exclusively plant based

Probiotics
Garden of Life
Symprove

Nutritional Testing and Consultations
Please contact the Nutrition Guru clinic for more information:
   https://www.thenutritionguru.co.uk/

References

All websites accessed June 2022

1. Set yourself up for success

'In 2018, researchers at Manchester Metropolitan University looked at 11 existing studies…': https://www.clinicalnutritionjournal.com/article/S0261-5614(18)32540-8/fulltext

'Certainly, if your diet is lacking in key nutrients or you are eating a diet that may cause inflammation, you are more likely to suffer low moods': https://www.sciencedirect.com/science/article/pii/S2666354619300171

2. Spot the signs of nutritional deficiency

'It's estimated that 40–50% of teenagers in the UK will have one or more nutrient deficiencies': https://www.gov.uk/government/collections/national-diet-and-nutrition-survey and https://www.hsis.org/wp-content/uploads/2020/12/HSIS_Dietary-Status-of-Teens_report_web.pdf

'Along with essential fats (the fats we can't make in our bodies), four of the most commonly occurring nutrient deficiencies in the UK are iron, magnesium, calcium and vitamin D, and again it's estimated teenagers are likely to be low in one or more of these at any time': https://www.gov.uk/government/collections/national-diet-and-nutrition-survey and https://www.hsis.org/wp-content/uploads/2020/12/HSIS_Dietary-Status-of-Teens_report_web.pdf

'There's little evidence to suggest gluten-free has any particular health benefits unless you are a coeliac or have a gluten intolerance': https://www.ncbi.nlm.nih.gov/pmc/articles/PMC6636598/, https://www.bmj.com/content/357/bmj.j2135 and https://celiac.org/about-the-foundation/featured-news/2017/05/study-finds-gluten-free-diet-adults-without-celiac-disease-may-increase-risk-cardiovascular-disease/

'The latest science shows that the artificial sweeteners in diet drinks and food disrupt our important gut microbiota and may lead to increased weight gain and type 2 diabetes': https://keck.usc.edu/looking-to-lose-weight-diet-drinks-might-not-be-the-sweet

-spot-according-to-new-usc-study/ and https://journals.plos.org/
plosmedicine/article?id=10.1371/journal.pmed.1003950

'Studies show that having breakfast improves concentration and
mood': https://www.ncbi.nlm.nih.gov/pmc/articles/PMC3737458/

'It's scientifically proven that food presentation makes food taste
better too': https://www.researchgate.net/publication/319592518
_Plating_and_Plateware_On_the_Multisensory_Presentation_of
_Food

3. Eat a rainbow and digestion 101

'Ideally, the goal is to eat between seven and ten fist-sized portions
of different fresh fruits and vegetables every day': https://www
.imperial.ac.uk/news/177778/eating-more-fruits-vegetables-prevent
-millions/

'In a study of people with chronic constipation, a daily exercise
regimen including 30 minutes of walking significantly improved
symptoms': https://journals.plos.org/plosone/article?id=10.1371/
journal.pone.0090193, https://go.gale.com/ps/i.do?p=AONE&u=anon
~6f9cfd12&id=GALE|A440635678&v=2.1&it=r&sid=googleScholar
&asid=81953978 and https://pubmed.ncbi.nlm.nih.gov/16028436/

'Would you believe that this affects up to 32% of the population, men
and women, to some degree': https://toiletanxiety.org/about.html

'You might also find anxiety-relieving techniques such as breathing
exercises, meditation or yoga, which you can learn and practise
from aps, will help to relieve digestive problems': Breethe (breathing
app), Insight Timer (meditation app) and 5 Minute Yoga or Yoga for
Beginners (yoga apps)

'There's a well-known yoga move called wind-relieving pose that
can shift bloating and gas': https://m.youtube.com/watch?v
=IvAx7q2LKqk and https://www.healthline.com/health/digestive
-health/how-to-fart#yoga-poses

4. Fats won't make you fat (but they will make you smart)

'Did you know that if you take away the water, 60% of our brains
are made of essential fats?': https://pubmed.ncbi.nlm.nih.gov
/20329590/

'Over time they can damage to the brain, affecting its ability to process
information in particular': https://www.ncbi.nlm.nih.gov/pmc/
articles/PMC6146358/

5. Balance your blood sugar for all-day energy

'In fact, studies have found links between antisocial behaviour and poor blood sugar control': https://onlinelibrary.wiley.com/doi/full/10.1002/pdi.854 and https://www.ncbi.nlm.nih.gov/pmc/articles/PMC4073202/

6. Good hydration

'Just a 1–2% drop in your body's water levels can reduce your attention span by 25%': https://www.ncbi.nlm.nih.gov/pmc/articles/PMC4207053/ and https://www.ncbi.nlm.nih.gov/pmc/articles/PMC6603652/

'It's been proved that drinking water slowly throughout the day makes you more hydrated than guzzling lots of water quickly': https://pubmed.ncbi.nlm.nih.gov/21997675/

'Researchers have discovered that even after you stop consuming caffeine, you may experience withdrawal symptoms': https://www.researchgate.net/publication/11511520_Caffeine_dependence_in_teenagers and https://www.ncbi.nlm.nih.gov/books/NBK430790/

'Caffeine takes a major toll on your sleep…': https://www.sciencedirect.com/science/article/abs/pii/S0271531713001528?via%3Dihub

'Teenagers aged between 13 and 17 are among the fastest growing population of caffeine users': https://www.ncbi.nlm.nih.gov/pmc/articles/PMC6136946/

'Given that energy drink use may cause behavioural problems and negatively impact mental health and well-being…': https://www.ncbi.nlm.nih.gov/pmc/articles/PMC4892220/

'A study following more than 4100 females and 3400 males for seven years as part of the Growing Up Today Study II…' https://www.ncbi.nlm.nih.gov/pmc/articles/PMC4180814/

7. What you eat can make you happier

'…all participants in the Australian Smiles Trial were medically diagnosed with moderate to severe depression': https://pubmed.ncbi.nlm.nih.gov/28137247/

'…the Helfimed Trial showed that a Mediterranean diet can improve mental health in adults suffering from depression': https://pubmed.ncbi.nlm.nih.gov/29215971/

'In one study students from Reading University were given 30g of freeze-dried wild blueberries in a flavonoid-rich drink': https://www.ncbi.nlm.nih.gov/pmc/articles/PMC5331589/

'...increasing your dietary intake of folate, zinc and magnesium may reduce depressive disorders': https://www.ncbi.nlm.nih.gov/pmc/articles/PMC4167107/#bib4

'...increasing dietary omega-3 fatty acids can reduce anxiety disorders': https://pubmed.ncbi.nlm.nih.gov/24196402/

'...studies have found that sticking to Mediterranean dietary patterns can reduce inflammation markers': https://pubmed.ncbi.nlm.nih.gov/21392646/ and https://www.bmj.com/content/369/bmj.m2382.short

'Oxidative stress is a bodily condition that happens when your antioxidant levels are low': https://www.sciencedirect.com/science/article/abs/pii/S1359644620301926

'A study conducted by University College London in 2019 showed that people who eat dark chocolate are less likely to be depressed': https://www.ucl.ac.uk/school-life-medical-sciences/news/2019/aug/people-who-eat-dark-chocolate-less-likely-be-depressed

'Dark red berries – particularly blueberries, but also blackberries and raspberries – have been shown to improve your memory and mood too': https://www.cambridge.org/core/journals/british-journal-of-nutrition/article/effect-of-4-weeks-daily-wild-blueberry-supplementation-on-symptoms-of-depression-in-adolescents/E8ED12AC48E936A4A8D6664B93AD6AA6 and https://www.research.manchester.ac.uk/portal/files/92960868/1_s2.0_S0889159118311954_main.pdf

'Vitamin D... prevents cancer development': https://www.cancer.gov/about-cancer/causes-prevention/risk/diet/vitamin-d-fact-sheet

'Research shows that having healthy levels of vitamin D, as well as taking a vitamin D supplement, can help keep your immune system healthy': https://www.ncbi.nlm.nih.gov/pmc/articles/PMC3166406/

'NHS UK recommends that everyone takes a Vitamin D supplement (10 mcg per day) throughout the winter months from September to April': https://www.nhs.uk/conditions/vitamins-and-minerals/vitamin-d/

'...check out the organisation Young Minds': https://www.youngminds.org.uk

'Studies have shown that simple handwashing can help prevent a large number of illnesses': https://adc.bmj.com/content/101/1/42

'Scientists are also finding more and more health benefits to having a quick blast of cold water in the shower': https://www.ncbi.nlm.nih.gov/pmc/articles/PMC4049052/

8. Going plant-based

'…add onion and garlic, as they have been shown to make iron (and zinc) more available to the body': https://pubmed.ncbi.nlm.nih.gov/20597543/

'…the Vegan Society is an inexpensive place to buy these from': https://www.vegansociety.com/shop/veg-1-supplements

'There are also other companies that produce excellent quality vegan supplements, including Cytoplan and Wild Nutrition': www.cytoplan.co.uk and https://www.wildnutrition.com

'Vegans and vegetarians need to consume 1.8 times more iron than omnivores': *Dietary Reference Intakes for Vitamin A, Vitamin K, Arsenic, Boron, Chromium, Copper, Iodine, Iron, Manganese, Molybdenum, Nickel, Silicon, Vanadium, and Zinc.* Institute of Medicine, Food and Nutrition Board. Washington, DC: National Academy Press, 2001.

9. Love the skin you're in

'Recent studies have looked at a number of skin conditions': https://www.ncbi.nlm.nih.gov/pmc/articles/PMC3970830/ and https://www.ncbi.nlm.nih.gov/pmc/articles/PMC7432353/ and https://www.sciencedirect.com/science/article/pii/S2666328722000281

'…we also have to think about our intake of sugar and fats': https://pubmed.ncbi.nlm.nih.gov/20620757 and https://lpi.oregonstate.edu/mic/health-disease/skin-health/essential-fatty-acids

'Researchers have also found that a diet high in omega-3 can make the skin less reactive to UV rays': https://onlinelibrary.wiley.com/doi/10.1111/j.1600-0625.2011.01294.x

'Wash your skin with a gentle cleanser or water after you exercise to ensure you wash away all the toxins you release': https://www.sciencedirect.com/science/article/pii/S0160412017319761#bb0020 and https://www.ncbi.nlm.nih.gov/pmc/articles/PMC3312275/

'In one study, acne sufferers on a 10-week low sugar diet saw a significant improvement in the appearance of their acne': https://pubmed.ncbi.nlm.nih.gov/17616769/ and https://www.ncbi.nlm.nih.gov/pmc/articles/PMC7847434/

10. Achieve a healthy weight for life

'Studies show that high added sugar consumption can lead to weight gain in teenagers and may also increase their risk of certain health conditions': https://www.ncbi.nlm.nih.gov/pmc/articles/PMC5133084/ and https://www.ncbi.nlm.nih.gov/pmc/articles/PMC4822166/

'Research also indicates that teenagers are more likely to consume sugary beverages if their parents do': https://www.ncbi.nlm.nih.gov/pmc/articles/PMC7311966/

'The Aggregate Nutrient Density Index (ANDI) is a scoring system that rates foods based on their nutrient content': https://www.drfuhrman.com/blog/128/andi-food-scores-rating-the-nutrient-density-of-foods

'...research has shown that consuming veggies can help teenagers reach and maintain a healthy body weight': https://www.cdc.gov/healthyweight/children/index.html and https://www.ncbi.nlm.nih.gov/pmc/articles/PMC5828430/

11. Gain weight and bulk up healthily

'...this is due to a process called protein synthesis, which means there's only a certain amount of protein your muscles can absorb in one sitting': https://www.ncbi.nlm.nih.gov/pmc/articles/PMC5828430/

'Weight-gain shakes are similar to other protein shakes, but they are very high in calories...': https://caliberstrong.com/blog/weight-gainer-mass-gainer-supplements/

'Recent studies have shown that young athletes consume two to three times the recommended amount of protein per day in their diet': https://www.ncbi.nlm.nih.gov/pmc/articles/PMC4590906/

'You can work out exactly how much protein you require with a simple calculation...': https://healthyeating.sfgate.com/much-protein-should-kid-day-6207.html

'For example, a 115 g serving of chicken, fish or beef provides 25–30g of protein, an egg provides 6 g and a glass of milk provides 8 g of protein': https://www.nutrition.org.uk/healthy-sustainable-diets/protein/?level=Health%20professional

12. Teenage hormone imbalance

'And a word about cortisol, which is commonly called the "stress hormone" and has a vital role in your body's response to stress': https://www.ncbi.nlm.nih.gov/pmc/articles/PMC6289691/

'Too much sugar leads to too much insulin': https://www.ncbi.nlm.nih
.gov/pmc/articles/PMC2764307/

'Higher levels of testosterone... raise the likelihood of PCOS': https://
www.ncbi.nlm.nih.gov/pmc/articles/PMC3846536/

'While excess sugar in the diet... may lower testosterone levels in men':
https://academic.oup.com/jcem/article/93/5/1834/2598879, https://
ec.bioscientifica.com/view/journals/ec/7/12/EC-18-0480.xml and
https://diabetesstrong.com/how-blood-sugar-levels-affect-your
-testosterone-sex-drive/

'Eating foods rich in essential fatty acids (such as mixed nuts, seeds,
oily fish, avocados, olive oil and seed oils) can make a big difference
to PMT symptoms': https://www.ncbi.nlm.nih.gov/pmc/articles/
PMC3033240/

'Research also shows a link between vitamin B6 and reduced depression and
irritability': https://www.ncbi.nlm.nih.gov/pmc/articles/PMC27878/ and
https://www.ncbi.nlm.nih.gov/pmc/articles/PMC4794546/

'Research suggests women who eat a diet rich in calcium have a 40%
lower risk of developing PMT': https://www.newscientist.com/article/
dn7515-calcium-rich-diets-may-prevent-pms/

'Diets low in vitamins B1, B2 and B6 are associated with a higher
occurrence of PMS': https://pubmed.ncbi.nlm.nih.gov/21346091/

'Women whose diet is rich in calcium are less likely to suffer PMS':
https://www.ncbi.nlm.nih.gov/pmc/articles/PMC7716601/, https://
pubmed.ncbi.nlm.nih.gov/9731851/, https://pubmed.ncbi.nlm
.nih.gov/17174829/ and https://jamanetwork.com/journals/
jamanetworkopen/fullarticle/2789711

'Phytoestrogens from foods such as tofu, edamame beans, lentils,
oats, barley, flaxseeds, sesame seeds, almonds and pistachios can
help balance your hormones': https://www.cambridge.org/core/
services/aop-cambridge-core/content/view/S0007114505001145

13. How to get more ZZZs

'So how much is enough sleep?': https://www.sleepfoundation
.org/how-sleep-works/how-much-sleep-do-we-really-need
and https://www.sleep.org/how-sleep-works/how-much-sleep
-children-need/

'Studies show that your body needs sunlight (blue light) as soon as
you rise and total darkness at night': https://www.sleepfoundation

.org/bedroom-environment/blue-light and http://healthysleep.med
.harvard.edu/healthy/science/how/neurophysiology

'If you sleep with the light on, your sleep will be shallow and you will
wake up frequently': https://pubmed.ncbi.nlm.nih.gov/24210607/,
https://www.ncbi.nlm.nih.gov/pmc/articles/PMC6751071/ and
https://www.cdc.gov/niosh/emres/longhourstraining/light.html

'Morning light suppresses melatonin, so your body wakes up, and it
also boosts serotonin': https://pubmed.ncbi.nlm.nih.gov/21459634/

'Growing evidence suggests that the gut microbiome can influence
sleep quality': https://www.ncbi.nlm.nih.gov/pmc/articles/
PMC6779243/ and https://journals.plos.org/plosone/article?id=10
.1371/journal.pone.0222394

'In fact, people who ate oily fish a couple of times a week had better
overall sleep': https://pubmed.ncbi.nlm.nih.gov/26847986/ and
https://pubmed.ncbi.nlm.nih.gov/24812543/

'Low levels of omega-3, present in oily fish, are also associated with
poorer sleep quality': https://www.mdpi.com/2072-6643/13/1/248

'Fibre provides the best fuel for our gut bacteria, which actually
makes the melatonin': https://www.ncbi.nlm.nih.gov/pmc/articles
/PMC3402070/ and https://ift.onlinelibrary.wiley.com/doi/10.1111
/1750-3841.14952

'Other research found that eating kiwi can improve sleep': https://
pubmed.ncbi.nlm.nih.gov/21669584/

14. Build a healthy relationship with food

'It takes about 20 minutes for the brain to realise that the stomach is
full': https://www.ncbi.nlm.nih.gov/pmc/articles/PMC5855475/

'There is plenty of help available online (for example, Beat... and
the Government of Western Australia's Centre for Clinical
Interventions...)': www.beateatingdisorders.org.uk and www.cci
.health.wa.gov.au/Resources/Looking-After-Yourself/Disordered
-Eating

16. All about anxiety

'...a 2001 study found optimal magnesium to be necessary for normal
sleep regulation too': https://pubmed.ncbi.nlm.nih.gov/11777170/

'Stress also depletes our B vitamins and studies show B vitamins help reduce our stress levels': https://www.ncbi.nlm.nih.gov/pmc/articles/PMC6770181/

'Research has shown that just a few minutes of daily meditation practice that includes deep rhythmic breathing, can reduce stress and anxiety, and help clear the mind': https://pubmed.ncbi.nlm.nih.gov/29616846/ and https://www.frontiersin.org/articles/10.3389/fpsyg.2021.724126/full

'We know that spending time in natural environments, like parks or woodlands or by lakes, can reduce stress': https://cpb-us-e1.wpmucdn.com/blogs.uoregon.edu/dist/e/12535/files/2015/12/ResponseNon-linear-28e9hbu.pdf

'...we know that exercise reduces anxiety too': https://www.ncbi.nlm.nih.gov/pmc/articles/PMC3632802/

'Students who exercise vigorously for 20 minutes a day, seven days a week, have been shown to achieve higher grades than students who don't': https://www.unh.edu/healthyunh/blog/physical-activity/2019/01/can-regular-exercise-improve-gpa

...as has being with friends and family: RE Adams, JB Santo and WM Bukowski, 'The presence of a best friend buffers the effects of negative experiences' in *Developmental Psychology*, 2011, 47(6), p. 1786. Available at: https://pubmed.ncbi.nlm.nih.gov/21895364/

17. Learning to love yourself

'In 2005, the US Government's National Science Foundation published an article that concluded the average person has somewhere between 12,000 and 60,000 thoughts every day': https://tlexinstitute.com/how-to-effortlessly-have-more-positive-thoughts/

'Health at every size (HAES) aims to promote self-care...: https://asdah.org/health-at-every-size-haes-approach/

Glossary

Additives substances added to food to preserve it or enhance its taste or appearance

Amino acid a type of molecule that combines to form a protein – there are nine essential ones that cannot be made by the body

Anorexia nervosa an eating disorder in which someone has an unhealthy obsession with losing weight and eats very little

Antioxidants substances that can prevent or slow damage to cells caused by free radicals

Bliss point where a particular food has just the right amount of saltiness, sweetness and richness to trigger a reward in your brain

Bulimia nervosa an eating disorder in which someone has an unhealthy obsession with losing weight, overeats and then purges by making themselves vomit

Chemicals a distinct compound or substance, especially one that has been artificially prepared

Circadian rhythms physical, mental and behavioural changes that follow a 24-hour cycle, primarily in response to light and dark

Depression a common mental disorder, characterised by persistent sadness and a lack of interest in previously rewarding or enjoyable activities – it can also disturb appetite, concentration and sleep

Diabetes a disease that affects your body's ability to produce or use insulin

Dopamine a 'happy' hormone

Endorphins	'happy' neurotransmitters and the body's natural painkillers
Essential fatty acids	fats that are essential to the diet because they cannot be made by the body – omega-3 is an essential fatty acid
Free radicals	unstable molecules in our body that can cause damage to our cells
GABA	a 'happy' neurotransmitter
Hormones	chemical substances that act like messenger molecules in the body
Insulin	a hormone that transports the energy produced by food to the cells – if you are diabetic and your body produces little or no insulin, too much sugar remains in your blood
Legumes	the seeds, usually in pods, of a family of plants – common edible legumes include peas, soya beans and peanuts
Melatonin	the sleep hormone
Metabolism	all the chemical processes in your body, especially those that cause food to be used for energy and growth
Microbiome	all the microbes – bacteria, fungi, protozoa and viruses – that live on and inside the human body, including in the gut
Neurotransmitters	the chemicals that form the body's cell-level messaging system – serotonin, dopamine, endorphins and GABA are all 'happy' neurotransmitters
Oestrogen	the female sex hormone that regulates the menstrual cycle
Omega-3	an essential fatty acid, found in, among other foods, oily fish and flaxseeds – vegans may need to take a supplement
Orthorexia nervosa	an eating disorder in which someone has an unhealthy obsession with eating healthily

Palpitations	heartbeats that suddenly become more noticeable – your heart may feel like it's pounding, fluttering or beating irregularly
Parabens	compounds used as preservatives in the pharmaceutical, cosmetics and food industries
Pharmaceuticals	any kind of drug or medicine used for medicinal purposes, for example paracetamol or cough syrup
Prebiotic foods	in your gut, they turn into 'good' bacteria
Probiotic foods	the non-digestible food parts that nourish the good bacteria in your gut
Progesterone	a sex hormone – it has an important role in the female menstrual cycle and males need it for the production of testosterone
Pulses	the edible seeds of plants in the legume family – they grow in pods, come in a variety of shapes, sizes and colours, and include beans, chickpeas and lentils
Resistance training	a form of exercise that involves making your muscles work against a weight (free weights, resistance bands, weight machines or your own body weight)
Satiety	the feeling of being full or satisfied by foods
Serotonin	a 'happy' neurotransmitter and the feel-good hormone
Testosterone	the male sex hormone
Tryptophan	an essential amino acid that is needed for the production of serotonin
Xenoestrogens	any natural or synthetic compound introduced into the body that mimics the effects of oestrogen or promotes its production

Index

5 x 5 approach   155, 170
80:20 rule   12–13, 16, 135, 149

acne   18, 53, 88–9, 92–3, 98, 112
alcohol   60–1, 120
amino acids   45, 67, 68, 82, 83–4, 108, 112, 131
anorexia nervosa   144, 146, 148
anti-inflammatory foods   91, 93–4
antioxidants   25, 26, 40, 43, 65, 73, 125
anxiety see stress and anxiety
artificial sweeteners   22, 36, 59

B vitamins   79–80, 87, 117, 124, 125–6, 131, 160
beans and legumes   26, 36, 38, 43, 51, 53, 68, 73, 80, 81, 82, 84, 91, 93, 103, 104, 108, 118, 121, 125, 131, 160
bloating   35–7, 38
blood sugar levels   45, 46, 47–9, 52, 53, 61, 68, 99, 101, 124, 129, 1134
body hair, excess   118, 121
bone health   19, 26, 57–8, 96
brain and gut connection   70–2, 77, 134
brain health   26, 40–3, 46, 47, 60, 70–2, 162
breakfast, importance of   23
breathing exercises   37, 38, 74, 92, 94, 122, 132, 154, 165

budget, eating on a   23
bulimia nervosa   144, 146, 148

caffeine   57–8, 59, 61, 90, 120, 130, 132
calcium   20, 79, 92–3, 125, 126, 131–2
carbohydrates   21, 43–6, 48, 53, 104–5, 127, 132, 133
casein   92, 108, 112
cheese   67, 68, 79, 92, 103, 104, 117, 118, 144
chicken and turkey   67, 93, 98, 103, 109, 117, 125, 131, 160
choline   40, 43, 81
coffee and tea   57, 58, 59, 61, 132
concentration   10, 13, 15, 16, 18, 20, 23, 41, 42, 43, 53, 54, 57, 96, 115, 123, 127, 130, 146
constipation   19, 34–5
cortisol   116, 118, 122
cow's milk   90, 92, 132

dairy products   22, 65, 71, 79, 81, 90, 92–3, 112, 126, 132
dark chocolate   65–6, 68, 77
dark circles under eyes   19
depression see mental health; mood swings; stress and anxiety
detox diets, fad   22
detox processes, natural   120, 123, 162
diabetes   50, 59, 98, 122

diets, weight loss *see* weight and health
digestion   32–6, 48, 55
dopamine/the motivator   67, 69, 77

eating disorders   144–9
eczema   93–4
eggs   22, 39, 40, 42, 43, 65, 67, 68, 102, 108, 109, 113, 116, 117, 118, 125, 144, 160
emotional eating   150–1
    5 x 5 approach   155, 157
    eating mindfully   154
    intuitive eating   155–6, 157
    keeping a food diary   152
    positive self-talk   153
    recognising emotional hunger   153
    triggers   144, 151, 154–5
    ways to feed your feelings   153–4
endorphins   68, 69, 77, 162, 165
endurance exercises   164
energy drinks   58–9, 98, 132
energy levels   43–4, 52, 53, 73, 93, 135–6, 142, 165
    see also blood sugar levels; sleep
Epsom salts   125, 133, 160
erectile dysfunction   115, 122
essential fatty acids   17, 124
exercise   33–4, 38, 69, 75, 89, 92, 94, 100, 103, 113, 120, 121, 124, 130, 133, 162–3
eye health   25, 28

fad diets   99–100, 146
fats, healthy   39–40, 41, 46, 48, 71, 87, 90, 99, 104, 124
    see also omega-3

fats, unhealthy/saturated   42, 90, 99
fermented food   36, 68, 71, 121
fibre, dietary   35, 38, 44, 51, 53, 61, 69, 98, 121, 124, 131, 135, 143
fight or flight response   32, 37, 118, 158
fish/shellfish   41–2, 46, 63, 65, 68, 91, 131, 132, 160
food as fuel   23–4
fruit and vegetables
    anti-inflammation   91
    blood sugar levels   49, 53
    colour in   25, 27–8, 38, 57, 91
    dark berries   43, 65, 77, 91
    hormone balance   120, 121
    leafy greens   65, 69, 73, 85, 91, 93, 117, 125, 131–2, 160
    mental health   62, 63, 64, 65, 66, 77

GABA   68, 69, 77
garlic   73, 77, 98
glucose   47, 59, 89
gluten-free foods   22
glycaemic index   51
goal setting   16, 101, 171–3
GPs/healthcare professionals   6, 74, 147, 159
gratitude, daily   168, 171
gut bacteria/microbiome   37, 44, 64, 70–2, 77, 89, 91, 99, 121, 131, 134

healthy habits   168–70, 171
heart health   19, 26, 28, 59
hormone imbalance
    delayed puberty   118

foods to help balance for
    boys 118, 126
foods to help balance for
    girls 116–17, 125–6
natural ways to regulate
    hormones 120, 121–2, 126
natural ways to regulate
    oestrogen 120
periods and PMS 114, 121, 123–6
signs in boys 115, 117
signs and causes in girls 114–16
weight gain 114, 116, 118,
    120, 122
hormones general 45, 46, 55, 61
hydration 32, 37, 38, 54–61, 87,
    90, 103, 120, 121, 133, 144,
    164

immune system 18, 28, 64, 73,
    74–5, 89, 127, 164
inflammation 64, 65, 89, 90,
    93, 124
insulin 121, 122
intuitive eating 155–6
iron 20, 80, 81

joint health 55
junk/fast food 13–15, 42, 71, 91,
    101, 113, 142–3
    see also sugar/sugary foods

kidney health 26, 120

liver health and function 98, 120,
    121, 124, 125
low glycaemic foods 51

magnesium 20, 125, 131, 133, 160
meal plans 105, 137–41

meat 65, 68, 91, 94, 103, 104,
    108, 117, 125, 160
    see also chicken and turkey
meditation 37, 38, 69, 74, 92, 94,
    131, 133, 160–1, 165
Mediterranean diet 62, 63, 64,
    71, 77
melatonin/sleep hormone 45, 46,
    61, 128, 130, 131, 132
mental health 18, 47
    food and feeling good 62–72,
        170
    gut health and immune
        system 70–5
    hydration 58, 59, 60, 61
    impact of exercise 162
    lack of sleep 127, 134
    see also eating disorders; emo-
        tional eating; stress and anxiety
mindful eating 154
mood swings 47, 53, 69–70,
    96, 124
    see also mental health
muscle growth 107, 109, 112,
    164

negative thinking 167, 174
nutritional deficiencies 17–20
nuts and seeds 24, 26, 38, 39,
    42, 43, 52, 53, 57, 65, 67, 68,
    69, 72, 80, 82, 84, 91, 98,
    99, 102, 103, 104, 108, 113,
    116, 121, 125, 131–2, 160

oestrogen 115, 116, 117, 119,
    121, 124
omega-3 41–2, 46, 63, 69, 77,
    80–1, 86, 90, 91, 116, 132
orthorexia nervosa 144–5

overeating, controlling   137–41, 143, 144
oxidative stress   64, 65

periods and PMS   114, 115, 118–19, 123–5
phytoestrogens   126
phytonutrients   25, 27, 28
plant-based diets *see* vegetarian and vegan diets
plant milks   79, 80, 82, 85, 90
polycystic ovary syndrome   118–19
poo/bowel movements   34–5, 37–8, 87, 120, 121
portion sizes   30–1, 142
poultry *see* chicken and turkey
probiotics and prebiotics   71–2, 77
progesterone   115, 117, 121
protein   42, 48, 82, 83–4, 98, 103, 108–12, 132, 133, 144
puberty, delayed   118

saliva production   33, 55
seasonal affective disorder   130
self-acceptance, physical   101, 166–7, 168, 171
self-care checklist   173
self-compassion   168
self-esteem checklist   75–6
self-soothing techniques   170
self-worth, increasing   170–1
serotonin/happy hormone   45, 46, 67, 69, 77, 130
shakes, protein   108
shakes, weight-gain   105–6
skin health   18, 25, 28, 53, 87–9, 96, 134
   and diet   89–91, 94

lifestyle habits   92, 94, 162
treating acne and eczema   92–4
sleep   45, 46, 58, 61, 96, 108, 123, 124, 127, 137
amount needed   128
bedtime routines   132–3
circadian rhythms   128–9
foods to help you sleep   131–2
gut/microbiome health   131
impact of noise and light   128, 133
melatonin   45, 46, 61, 128, 130, 131, 132
mental health   127, 134, 160
screen displays   131, 133
SMART goals   171–3
smoothies, drinking   56–7, 61, 64, 91, 93
snacking   23, 52, 102, 133
social media   159, 171
socialising and food   134, 135
stress and anxiety   32, 33, 37, 38, 68, 74–5, 89, 92, 115, 118, 122, 124, 125, 144–5, 154, 170
finding some head space   161
five-step exercise   158–9
foods to help lessen   160
magnesium and B vitamins   160, 165
physical activity   162–4
survival guide   165
when it becomes a problem   159
yoga, mindfulness and meditation   160–1, 165
stretching exercises   35, 37, 38, 124, 164
sugar-free/diet drinks   22

sugar/sugary food and drinks   47,
    49–51, 53, 56, 58–9, 89, 90,
    121–2, 132, 135–6
    see also blood sugar; glucose
sunlight, morning   129, 130
supplements, dietary   82–3, 86,
    108, 109, 112, 126, 132

testosterone   117, 118, 121–2
tiredness/fatigue   18, 73, 118,
    124, 154
tofu   39, 80, 81, 103, 108, 116,
    126, 160
toilet, going to   34–5, 37–8, 87,
    120, 121
tooth health   53, 59, 98
trigger foods   144, 151
tryptophan   21, 45, 67, 68, 131, 132

vegetarian and vegan diets   21–2,
    78–9, 112
    food supplements   82–3, 86,
        126, 132
    getting the right nutrients
        79–86
    protein-combining   83–4
    sleep-promoting foods   132
vitamin A   79–80, 87
vitamin B   117
vitamin B1   125
vitamin B2   125
vitamin B6   124, 125, 131
vitamin B12   80, 125–6
vitamin C   87, 117
vitamin D   20, 74, 82, 117, 118,
    126, 130

vitamins and minerals
    general   18–20, 42–3, 55,
        56, 64, 79–82, 98
    supplements   82–3, 86, 108,
        109, 112, 126, 132

weight and health   22, 30, 44, 53,
    59, 127
    avoiding sugary food   99
    best weight-gain foods   103–5,
        108–9, 113
    exercise   100, 106–7, 113
    goal setting   101
    hormones and weight
        gain   114, 116, 118, 120
    nutrient rich foods   98, 100,
        101
    weight-gain meal plan and
        shakes   105–6
    why diets don't work   95–6,
        99–100, 101, 141
whole grains   38, 43, 44,
    45–6, 49, 53, 65, 81, 89,
    91, 98, 100, 102, 103,
    104, 118, 121, 125, 131,
    143, 160
wind/flatulence   35, 37, 38

xenoestrogens   119–20, 126

yoga/Pilates   37, 69, 74, 94,
    122, 124, 131, 133, 160–1,
    165
yoghurt   84, 85, 104, 118, 125

zinc   81, 87, 94, 117, 118

About the author

Tina Lond-Caulk is a Registered Nutritionist with over 20 years' experience, including working with a number of high-profile integrated medical practices in Harley Street and the world-renowned Lanserhof Medical Clinic. In addition to her first-class BSc Honours degree in Nutrition, she has post-graduate training in behavioural psychology and eating disorders. She is now Director of her own health clinic, the Nutrition Guru, where she leads a team of expert nutritionists, eating disorder dieticians and counsellors. She is a regular speaker at schools and for corporate wellness events.

Tina is passionate about sharing her knowledge and wholeheartedly believes that nutrition education is essential for young people. She developed the Food for Life programme for schools in 2009 and has worked with thousands of young people to educate and empower them to understand the importance of nutrition and healthy lifestyle choices, and how they can positively impact every aspect of well-being.

The goal of the Nutrition Guru is to help shape the health, well-being and self-esteem of current and future generations. For more information, please see: http://www.thenutritionguru.co.uk/